Escape from Communist Hungary

by

Zsuzsanna Bozzay

Published in 2013 by FeedARead.com Publishing –
Arts Council funded

Cover photo by Peter Vallelly

A CIP catalogue record for this title is available from the British Library.

Acknowledgements

With grateful thanks to my husband Michael,
Delia Creedy, Kathy Horton and Christine Turner for their suggestions and help with correcting the text.

Chapter 1.

Life under communism.

At the end of the war in 1945 Hungary became part of the Russian buffer zone. In fact it was now under Russian occupation, as decided by Churchill, Roosevelt and Stalin at the Yalta Conference. Hungary was once again punished for being on the wrong side of the war.

There were food shortages just like in other European countries but there was no rationing as in England. People had to queue for basic foods and often when they had reached the end of the queue there was nothing left to buy. We had all lost a lot of weight and felt exhausted after enduring months of bombings, with little sleep and constant worry. Many members of my mother's Jewish family disappeared in the concentration camps although her brother *Feri* had, by some miracle, just managed to survive. He was found by a woman doctor when the concentration camp was liberated by the Russians. She noticed a flicker of movement in his eyes as he lay barely alive among a pile of dead bodies. She lifted him up and carried him out. He was suffering from typhus and was skin and bone, so emaciated that even his own wife did not recognise him when she tried to find him in the hospital. My mother accompanied her and recognised him from his big blue eyes. He recovered but it took a long time. We all felt lucky to be alive.

My father returned to work at the office of a firm making hunting rifles and ammunition, called the *Vadásztöltény Gyár* and gradually life returned to normal.

We spent a few weeks during the summer at *Csillaghegy*, a holiday resort a few miles north of Budapest with three large swimming pools and extensive grounds where I could run around unsupervised and play with other children. My parents rented a room near the entrance in the main building which looked out on a large shared terrace with tables and chairs. Underneath this terrace there was a restaurant where live music was performed on the stage in the evenings. My mother thought that I had quite a good singing voice and encouraged me to enter a competition but when I stood on the stage I was so terrified that hardly any sound came out however hard she encouraged me. I could not understand why I wasn't given a microphone. My father came after work every day as it could be easily reached from the city. I spent the happiest times of my childhood in this place where I had so much freedom playing with other children in the terraced gardens full of dahlias and roses or swimming in one of the three pools and later I often dreamed that I was back there. It was my paradise.

Once I nearly drowned when I went into the deep end of one of the pools by holding on to the rail along the side and I slipped off the shallow ledge into the deep water. I was trying desperately to get hold of the ledge when a man standing by the side of the pool noticed me and pulled me out. I don't think I told my parents of my mishap otherwise they would not have allowed me to go into the pool unsupervised again.

I started ballet lessons when I was five and at the end of the year took part in a theatre performance as a fairy in a short pink sequined tutu with several tulle petticoats. I had to dance around the bed of a sleeping girl and throw rose petals on her after she sang a solo with her teddy bear. I was also the female 'Compère' in a pale blue dress. I had to recite a short introduction to the programme in front of the curtains. At the end of the performance all the children stood in a row, and instead of taking a bow they drank a glass of milk. We were all reminded to bring a glass but I did not listen so at the rehearsal they gave me the milk can instead, which upset me very much. I threw it down into the orchestra pit shouting that fairies do not drink out of a milk can. The conductor demanded that I was immediately given a glass.

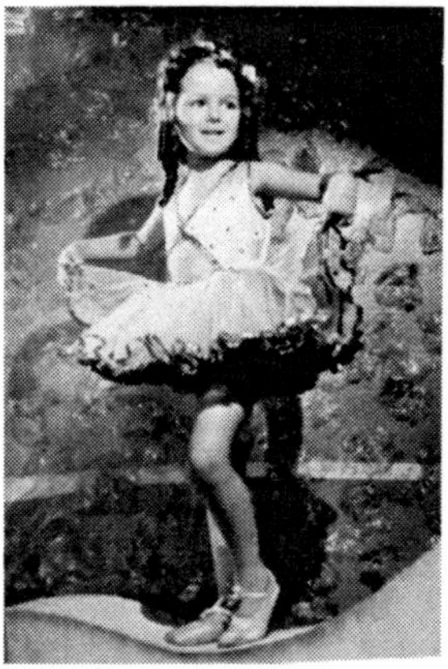

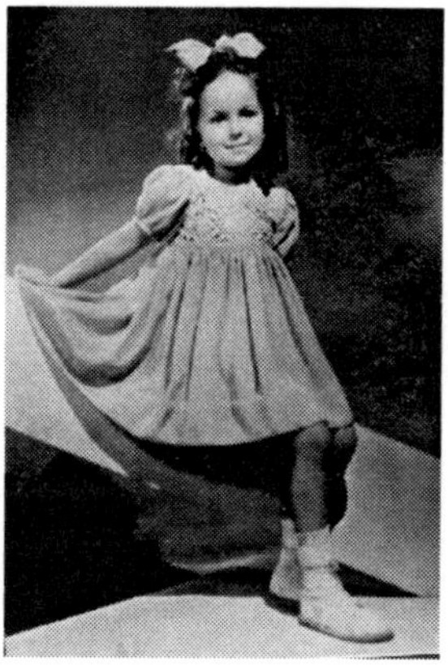

In September 1947, at the age of six, I started primary school in Budapest which is the usual age in Hungary. Luckily that year school started just after my birthday, otherwise I would have had to wait a whole year. My grandfather often accompanied me to school as we walked around the *Lövölde Tér*, the tree lined 'Shooters Square'. It probably took ten to fifteen minutes to walk to school from *Bajza utca* 2 (pronounced Boiza ootsa) where we lived on the sixth floor. I have very little memory of my early school days except for the fact that we were not allowed to lean on the desk with our elbows, instead we had to sit with both hands clasped behind our backs to stop fidgeting and to encourage good posture. The teacher would bang my elbow hard on the surface if she found it on the desk which was very painful. I have a photograph taken at the end of the year, in 1948. I am standing at the right hand end of the second row with my hair parted in the middle and ribbons above my ears holding curls of plaits. The class of eighteen girls assembled in the small tarmac covered playground for the photograph which is framed with a rhyming communist slogan above and underneath, 'Produce more for a better life! Study hard and you'll go far!' We hated these communist slogans.

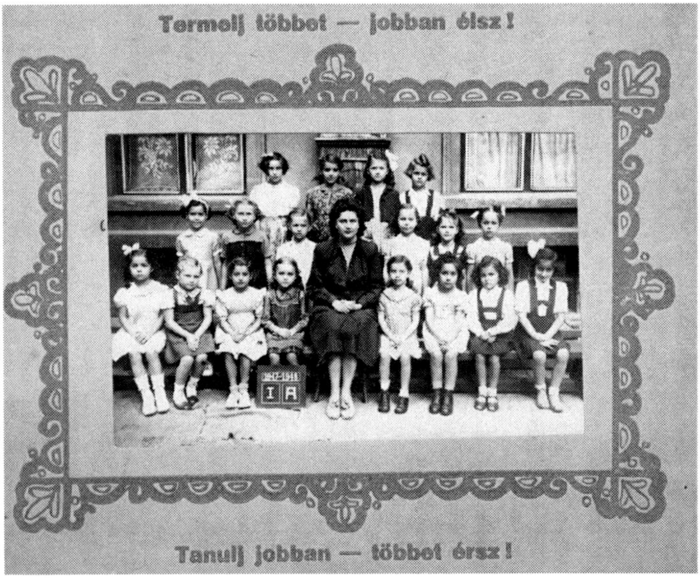

In 1947 a coalition government was formed after the elections. The Communists had very few votes, which did not please the occupying Russian forces, who wanted the Communists to be in power. It took two years to achieve their aim by starting a reign of terror; deporting, imprisoning and executing leaders of the opposition as well as ordinary people. My father's brother was imprisoned for political activities with the Smallholders Party and held in the headquarters of the secret police, the AVO on *Andrássy út 60*, which is now the Terror House, a museum and memorial for the victims of communism who were tortured and died there. My mother had a cousin who was a high ranking communist official there and she persuaded him to release her brother-in-law. Later this cousin committed suicide when he realised that communism was not what he thought it was.

People had to be careful of what they said in public places in case they were accused of being anti-communist and thrown into prison. We were frightened if there was a knock at the door, especially late at night in case it was the secret police. If we happened to be listening to the BBC we not only switched off the radio, but we also changed to a different station, because listening to western radio was punishable and could result in a prison sentence. But we knew that the only reliable source of news came from the BBC World Service. People could be imprisoned for no apparent reason, maybe because someone with a grudge against them accused them of being 'enemies of the people' and that was enough for the secret police to call and take them away. These were the methods of intimidation developed in the Soviet Union which were used by Lenin and continued by Stalin who invented the term an 'enemy of the people' to eliminate dissidents and hold people in terror, fearing for their lives.

It was not possible to get a passport in Hungary during communist times and without it we could not leave the country, but my mother was determined to escape from the regime and to go to London where her brother lived. The only way to get out of Hungary was to walk through the border illegally which was very dangerous, especially crossing into Austria in the west where the border was well guarded. But apparently it was easier to cross from Czechoslovakia into Austria. The border between Hungary and Czechoslovakia was not especially well guarded in the east, close to the Ukrainian border, as most people did not think of crossing there from one communist country into another. This gave my parents the idea that we should try our luck there but it took a long time to make the preparations. My father was reluctant to leave all his belongings behind unlike my mother who had no such attachment to possessions. One day when we lived in the flat on the sixth floor during the war, she found an unexploded bomb in the hall, which had fallen through the roof. She often said that she wished it had exploded and blown up all our belongings so that my father would not be held back by them. But they meant a lot to him. He had inherited his mother's books, silver, paintings and furniture. He had worked hard for the rest of our property. My mother was not attached to worldly goods; she knew that most things could be purchased. But there were some things like our dining room furniture which could not be bought because they were designed by my father's brother. It was very unusual furniture made of dark wood carved in an old Hungarian style, which was quite unique. So my mother had an idea. She met and made friends with an English couple at the British Embassy called Zena and John. She sometimes invited them for a meal. Zena could never understand why Hungarians would sprinkle poppy seeds on their nice clean pasta and make it look 'dirty'. When Zena and John were returning home to England my mother asked them if they would take our furniture as their own and they agreed, but unfortunately the plan failed. The furniture was confiscated because it was so typically Hungarian that the authorities did not believe it belonged to an English couple. It was put into store and we did not see it for several years.

Without our furniture we moved into two furnished rooms on the first floor of a villa in *Izso utca*. It was part of a flat that once belonged to a friend called *Serényi Aranka*, a Jewish lady, who left for London before the war. There was another family living next door and we had to share the kitchen and bathroom with them, but it was only a temporary measure as my parents were planning their escape.

One of the rooms had beautiful yellow English damask covering on the walls and in the other there was a typically Hungarian, six foot high free standing stove covered with green tiles and had a large shiny copper samovar on the top. The first room opened to the large balcony, with a wide stone balustrade with plant pots and a statue of a crouching lady on one corner. The balcony was big enough for a table and some chairs. Little ants came up from ground level which I enjoyed observing for hours on end. I was fascinated by their orderly marching and the way they carried crumbs much larger than themselves. They would also take away any ants that were accidentally damaged by me.

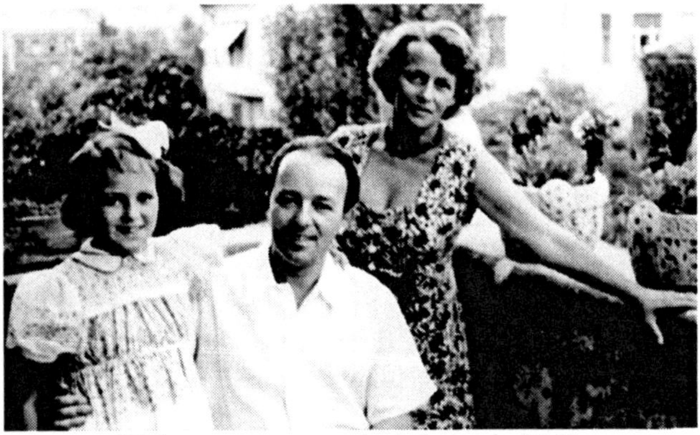

With my parents on the balcony in 1949

From the balcony I could also watch for my father coming home from work and when I saw him I would run down as fast as I could to meet him. On seeing me he would squat down and I ran into his wide open arms and he lifted me up high. I thought that my father was all powerful and I adored him as most little girls adore their fathers. He had endless patience teaching me things, such as how to ride a bicycle, holding on to the back of my neck for balance and how to mend all kinds of things. I thought the world of him and in my eyes he could do no wrong.

The following September I started the second year of primary school in the Notre Dame on the *Dózsa György út* near the *Városliget* (City Park). It was one of the last remaining religious schools and there I made friends with

Darányi Magdi, who lived on the opposite side of the road. She had a younger brother called *Dudi*, who was not yet at school and we spent many afternoons playing happily in their large garden. We used to collect ladybirds sheltering under leaves in the rain and put them in matchboxes. Our mothers became lifelong friends. Their parents were from a highly aristocratic family which was a disadvantage and something to hide.

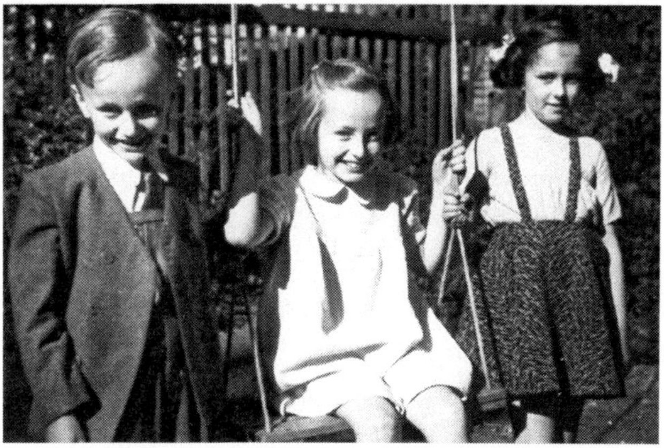

Dudi, Magdi and me in their garden.

An even greater disadvantage was the fact that Magdi's aunt Ilona had been married to *István (Stephen)*, the Vice-Regent and son of the Regent, *Horthy Miklós.* István was a pilot during the Second World War and was killed in the Ukraine, not during action by the Russian enemy, but apparently by the Germans for being friendly with the British and for trying to negotiate joining Hungary with the Allies. In 1944 near the end of the war Horthy Miklós was deposed by the Germans for negotiating a cease fire with the Soviets and sent into exile. They put the Arrow Cross party in power who were Nazi sympathisers.

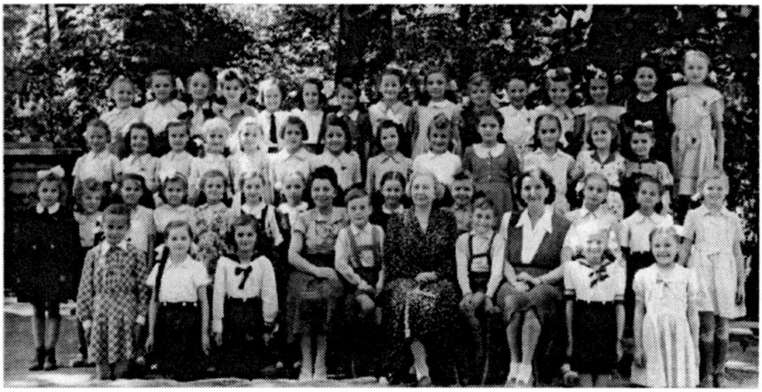

There were forty four girls and two little boys in the class in the Notre Dame School as can be seen on the above photograph. I was standing in the top row, sixth from the left next to my friend Magdi. At the end of the school year in 1949, I made my First Holy Communion wearing a short white dress and then I had to kneel on the cold stone floor of the church with the other members of my class. Afterwards we assembled outside the church and I recited a poem to the whole gathering. I remember the holy picture I was given as a memento, with a young child Jesus carrying a lamb on his shoulder with the quotation from Scripture underneath: 'My yoke is easy and my burden is light'.

At that time there was a possibility of Jewish people emigrating to the newly established country of Israel and my mother considered going there but one of the requirements was being able to speak Hebrew. My parents started to learn Hebrew but for some reason the idea was abandoned. Maybe they found it too difficult but I think that my mother really wanted to live in England and not in Israel. She wrote to her brother to ask if he could find them a position with a wealthy family in the country where they needed a cook and a chauffeur. Of course he could not find any such vacancy, but she carried on planning to live in England. When she decided something she would not give up and she was not afraid of new challenges. It takes a very special kind of person to leave all their possessions behind and move to a new country but she was not frightened by the prospect. It took all her powers of persuasion to convince my father of her plan. He was a staunch Hungarian, with very deep roots in Hungarian culture, had no talent for languages and found it hard to imagine living anywhere else, but eventually she had her way as she always did.

They decided to leave separately, because it was safer and less obvious that we were escaping the country. My father was going to follow later because we knew of several families who had lost everything when they were caught at the border trying to escape. They had nowhere to live when they came out of prison. In Budapest having a flat was very important and it still is. My father promised to follow us when he was sure that we were safe and smuggle out what valuables he could in the form of diamonds in his pocket. My mother said she would to ring him from Vienna as soon as we arrived.

Chapter 2.
The escape.

My parents were careful to keep their plans a secret and when finally the time came to leave there were no tearful good-byes and we did not pack any clothes for the journey. I had no idea where we were going or the reason for it. I was only just eight years old and I asked no questions, knowing that even if I did my mother was not in the habit of giving me explanations.

One morning we went to the Eastern Railway Station near our home, the *Keleti PU* as my mother jokingly called it, (pronouncing it 'poo', which has connotations in English, but not in Hungarian) and bought tickets to a town in the east of Hungary. Without any luggage we did not appear to be leaving the country. At the station we said good bye to my father, who went to work as usual. My mother and I boarded the train and at lunchtime she unpacked some pieces of cold chicken thighs fried in bread crumbs. It was one of my favourites.

It was late afternoon by the time we arrived at the border town of *Sátoraljaújhely* near Czechoslovakia and close to the Ukrainian border. At the station we were met by a guide who knew the terrain and offered to smuggle us across the border for a fee. We followed him through the quiet town, until we reached open fields. We continued through a forest climbing up a slope and reached the top of the hill where he showed us to a small shepherd's hut. There was straw on the floor and a piece of sacking for a door, which was flapping in the cold October wind. There were three other couples already settled in there.

'Make yourselves comfortable, but be very quiet. I'll be back after dark and show you the way across the border,' the guide said as he left.

We settled down on the straw, not daring to talk to the others. I soon fell asleep, I was exhausted.

It was pitch dark with no moon or stars in the sky when the guide returned and it was beginning to rain. A dog was barking in the distance and when my mother woke me up I wondered where we were going at such a late hour. We could hardly see our guide as he led us across the fields. My mother had to drag me along so that we did not fall behind and my tired feet were squelching in the soft mud. At times I felt I could go no further, but eventually it started getting lighter and in the distance we could see a railway station. We were in Czechoslovakia.

Our guide, who spoke Slovak, bought us tickets to the nearest town, *Kassa* and told us to wait on the platform. I was pleased when the train arrived and at last I could sit down to rest. It was not long before we arrived in *Kassa*, now called *Kosice*, where my mother found a taxi to take us to the address of our relatives.

The elderly lady who opened the door was very surprised to see us but when my mother explained who we were, she welcomed us in. She was a distant relative of my father and she lived with her sister. They gave us some food and drink while my mother told her why we had come. They allowed us to sleep on their settee for one night but we did not want to stay any longer and impose on their hospitality.

The next morning we went back to the station where my mother bought some food for the journey and tickets to *Pozsony*, which today is called *Bratislava*. She told me that I had to be very quiet, as some people in Czechoslovakia were not too fond of Hungarians. We worried in case we were questioned by the police or officials on the train about the reason for our journey but no one checked us. The train journey was very long and exhausting; we were travelling for about ten hours going towards the west. When we arrived, my mother found a room to rent and we settled down.

We spent about a week in *Pozsony*. It had been a Hungarian city for many centuries before the Treaty of Trianon in 1920 when Hungary was carved up and lost much of its territories for being on the wrong side of the war the last time, so my mother was able to find people who spoke Hungarian quite easily and she asked around trying to find someone to take us across the border to Austria. She was advised to go to the Synagogue to be put in touch with a guide who would help us to freedom and there she was given the address of a Hungarian speaking man who was to be our guide. He told her to meet him outside the Synagogue at ten o'clock the following evening. There were about ten people waiting outside in the dark. When the guide arrived we followed him out of the city, across the bridge and about half an hour later reached the outskirts. There were no more buildings here, just open fields. Pozsony is practically on the Austrian border. We kept walking along narrow paths and across fields for about another hour, meeting no one in the dark.

It was a cold, peaceful, moonlit night, not a sound could be heard as we sat down to rest in a field of corn, only about fifty metres from the Austrian border. We were almost in Austria, as the guide explained the next move.

'I am going to go ahead across the border, and when I've arrived and it's safe for you to follow I'll make a sound like an owl. You'll follow me one at a time, on all fours, so that if anyone sees you from a distance they'll think that you are dogs.' As he said this we saw two tiny figures on the horizon.

'Don't worry! They are only smugglers returning from Austria,' he said and carried on talking without lowering his voice. There was no wind and his voice travelled far in the still air. The two distant figures heard it, started walking in our direction and to our surprise we saw that they were not smugglers but carrying rifles on their backs. When they reached us they pointed their rifles at us and started shouting.

'Hands up! Hands up!'

We had to raise our arms, while they searched us for weapons and we wondered if we were going to be shot or arrested. We were terrified. I expect that the border guards were also terrified as there were only two of them against twelve of us and they didn't know if we were carrying any weapons. All my mother could say in Czech was '*Tohleje moje dcera*,' which means 'This is my daughter', and she kept repeating these words.

We were marched back to the road, bundled into a van and taken to a detention centre where the men were separated from the women. My mother and I were shown into a large room where several mothers and children were held. The conditions here were not as bad as in a prison cell. I remember seeing a young child having an epileptic fit as he lay on the floor with foaming mouth. It was a very frightening scene.

After we had been given something to eat and drink we were ushered into another small van to be handed over to the Hungarian authorities. My mother was more frightened of the Hungarian police than the Czech so when no one was looking, she decided to take off her gold watch and forced it into a small gap in the floor. After we were transferred at the border she saw the Czech guard searching the van hoping to find some valuables and she thought that he had probably found her watch.

We were taken to Szombathely, the town where both my mother's grandparents and my father's grandmother are buried. We were thrown into a cold bare cell with iron bars across the broken window. The iron beds had rusty bare springs, no mattress and no blankets. It was freezing cold and every few hours a prison guard came in and shouted at us calling us imperialist pigs and other nasty names, so that we could not get any sleep.

The next day my mother and I were taken to an orphanage and then I had to say good bye to her. There were three children sleeping in the one bed and I remember sitting on the bed while one of the girls was telling rude jokes. Before she was taken back to prison my mother managed to ask one of the women there to send a telegram to my father telling him that she was taken into custody and asking him to come and collect me. He arrived the next day and took me home to Budapest.

My mother later told me about the terrible overcrowded conditions in the prison cell where she was kept. There were more than ten women in a tiny cell and she had to share a small hard bed with another woman. They were locked in all day, given very little food or drink and it was very miserable, cold and dirty. She was taken in front of a Police Chief and interrogated about why she tried to cross the border illegally.

'I am very sorry!' she said. 'I had an argument with my husband, I lost my head and I decided to leave him, I was just walking aimlessly and I'd lost my way and didn't realise that I was so close to the Austrian border. I do love my country and I love communism, I just made a mistake.'

She had put on a very convincing act; she was a very good actress. It seemed that she had managed to convince him. At the same time my father consulted a lawyer, who was a good friend of his, and he intervened on her behalf. As a result of this her imprisonment was reduced to one month.

A week or so after I arrived home I became very ill with a high temperature and a violent headache. It started one evening while my father was talking on the telephone and I kept jumping on the sofa and he said that this was the reason for my headache. As I kept complaining and was obviously ill, a doctor was called, who thought at first that I might have meningitis and recommended that I should be admitted to hospital. Meningitis and polio have the same initial symptoms and to distinguish between them I had to undergo some tests. One of these was a very painful lumbar puncture. I had to sit on the edge of an examination couch and my back was bent over, then a large needle was inserted into my spine between the vertebrae to draw some fluid off. The result of the test confirmed that I had contracted poliomyelitis.

I was put in an isolation ward.

Chapter 3.

Grandparents.

My parents fell in love in 1931 when my father Emil was nearly twenty one and attending the Technical University of Budapest and my mother Mimi was twenty seven. She was supporting her elderly parents by working as a secretary for a firm selling parquet floors.

Her father Adolf had been a successful businessman in his younger days with a very good income as a tea and coffee merchant. He had a shop in the centre of Budapest on one of the large boulevards. He wore elegant top hats, had a pointed curly moustache and smoked expensive cigars. He often travelled on business to Vienna or Fiume on the Adriatic coast, but he had to give up work in his sixties as he was suffering from angina.

Her mother was always called Lotti but her real name was Sarolta, (pronounced Sharolta) the Hungarian for Charlotte. She was well educated, rarely wore any make up and was not very interested in cooking or housework, instead she liked to read, study and translate poetry from French or English and she also made exquisite lace pieces using bobbins. She walked with a stick and had a limp due to a childhood accident caused by a local doctor cutting through her Achilles tendon while lancing a boil. She received her teaching diploma from the *Veres Palné College* in Budapest, which was the first college that opened for women in Hungary in 1870 only three years before she was born. Lotti gave private lessons in French and German, but she could teach other subjects such as history and literature as well. Adolf and Lotti were both Jewish although not orthodox and this may have been the reason why she never taught in a school. Times were hard especially for Jews and they decided to emigrate to Paris. In 1921 they sent their eighteen year old son Imre, followed three years later by my mother Mimi. But Adolf became ill and when they realised that they were not able to manage on their own, they had to ask my mother to return. She had spent three very happy years in Paris with her brother but being a dutiful, loving daughter she returned home, although with a heavy heart. It is often a daughter's duty to look after her parents and she accepted this without a question. But she was always longing to go and live close to her brother, which eventually turned out to be London.

By 1930 both my parents were living in the same building, in *Rákóczi út 61*. This wide road, named after a national hero, is one of the important boulevards that lead from the Eastern Railway Station, the *Keleti PU,* to the centre of the city with many large shops and offices in beautiful buildings from the late nineteenth century with spacious flats on each of the four floors. There are many similar large tenement buildings in Budapest, all built at the turn of the century, usually with a large carved wooden door opening from the street onto a short covered passage from where there is a staircase to the upper floors and a central courtyard open to the sky allowing plenty of light in. Circling the courtyard there are wrought iron balconies on each floor, decorated with flowers and plants with entrances to the individual flats, about four to six on each floor. My mother's family had recently moved from a second floor flat in number 24 on the same road to a ground floor flat in this house because her father could not climb the stairs any more.

My father Emil lived on the first floor with his mother Margit, whom he called *Mucó* (pronounced Mootso), his brother *Cincó* (pronounced Tsintso) who was two years younger and a maid, *Böske.*

Adolf, my grandfather, was very interested in all modern innovations. He had a telephone which he had installed when he opened the Raphael Photographic Studio in his previous flat. Having a telephone was quite rare in the 1920s and 30s. Margit, my father's mother married very young and because the marriage was not happy, she divorced her husband and left the city of *Szombathely* near the Austrian border to start a new life in the capital in 1923. This was a very brave step in those days with two young boys and no support from her family. At first she could only earn a meagre living by dressmaking and almost starved, but after she took her book of published poems to the editor of the popular daily paper, the *Pesti Napló,* she became a highly respected and well known journalist and writer thanks to his support and encouragement.

She sometimes asked if she could use Adolf's telephone and so they became good friends. She must have looked on him as a father figure because she used to greet him by kissing him on both cheeks. He was in his late sixties, a distinguished looking gentleman with an aquiline nose and thick white hair. He had a room with its own entrance which was sublet to a young man called *Sándor Dajkovich* who was producing a book called The Encyclopaedia of Hungarian Women. (*Magyar Nők Lexicona* published in 1931). My grandfather Adolf became involved with the work and helped him with the financial side. Women who wanted to be included in the book had their pictures taken, wrote a short autobiography and then paid a sum of money which Adolf collected. There were several agents who visited famous ladies and interviewed them for inclusion in the Encyclopaedia. It was a very good money making idea. Adolf suggested that they ask a famous woman writer to write an introduction, as this would attract people to buy the book. They asked my grandmother Bozzay Margit to be the editor. This meant a substantial royalty payment for her when the book was published and purchased not only by the women included in it, but their friends and relations too. Margit was overjoyed to have this work and maybe it was to repay this kindness that she decided to take my mother on holiday to the Austrian Alps together with her friend *Ila* and Ila's daughter, the young *Ági.* In the photograph taken on this holiday Margit, the tallest figure, is standing behind *Ági* who is next to my mother wearing a beret. The girl on the right is probably a local guide. The Encyclopaedia, as well as this holiday is mentioned in Margit's second autobiographical novel entitled Labour and Love *(Kenyér és Szerelem)* which was published in 1936, although she did not acknowledge the source of the commission.

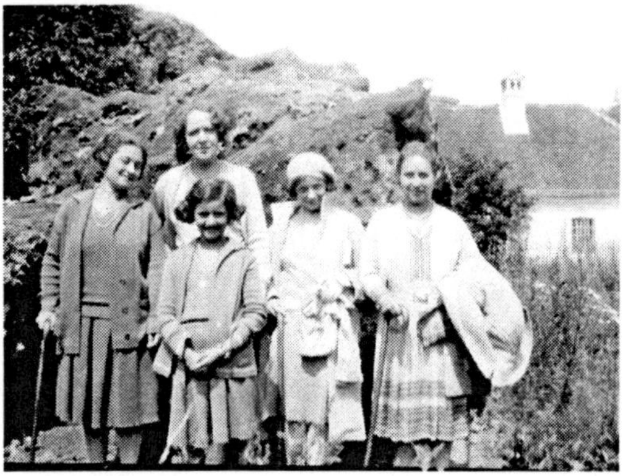

As well as being a columnist of the daily paper, the *Pesti Napló,* she was also an 'agony aunt' and produced a women's page for the paper. She gave advice to women and had very modern ideas. She believed in women's independence and their right to work although she felt that they were disadvantaged by the biology of their bodies. She was very popular and successful but she still found it difficult to make ends meet. Every month she divided her earnings into 30 envelopes, after setting aside the rent and every day her maid Böske, who came with her from the country, took one envelope to buy food. Böske did all the cooking, the washing and the cleaning, while Margit sat at her desk all day and most of the night, writing. The first book she wrote was an autobiographical novel, The Fifteen Year Old Wife, (*Tizenöt éves feleség)* which was published in 1936 and had several reprints. Although she was just 17 when she married, she wanted to stress that she was too young. She said to my mother, 'Everyone who reads my book will know how much I have suffered!'

My grandfather Adolf had angina since he was in his forties and my mother lived in constant fear of him dying.

She loved her father dearly; he was a very warm hearted generous man. He would give away his last coat to anyone who needed it. Every afternoon he went to the café to play dominoes and chat with his friends. Poor old ladies came to sell matches and he always bought some, even when he did not need them. He was always trying to make people laugh and was cheerful even though he was unable to work and had frequent angina attacks. Mimi used to make sure that his arm was not above his head when he slept because that would put a strain on his heart. But in the end nothing could be done to save him. Mimi and Lotti were with him in hospital when he died. He was 66 years old. Mimi thought her life had ended and she sobbed and screamed uncontrollably. But my grandmother Lotti remained calm and bore her loss with fortitude. When they returned from the hospital Emil visited them and tried to console Mimi. This was how their relationship started in January 1931.

Emil's mother Margit was quite friendly towards Mimi before her father died, but when the relationship between her son and Mimi became more serious, she put every obstacle in their way. She did not think that Mimi was good enough for her son, she was too poor, too old and she was also Jewish. In Hungary at that time there were laws which forbade Jews and Christians to marry or even to have a relationship. Margit said that she would rather see Emil laid out dead in front of her than to see him marry my mother. She was very possessive. Surely there could be nothing worse for a mother than to see her child dead.

Margit had other plans for the future; she was saving

up to live with her sons in a suburban villa surrounded by a large garden. She was completely wrapped up in their lives and, even though she had several serious relationships, she never married again. To her credit she made sure that her sons kept in touch with their father who also remained single for the rest of his life. I think that he deeply regretted his behaviour towards Margit and never stopped loving her.

Chapter 4.

Mimi.

My mother was born in March 1904 and was called Miriam which was later shortened to Miri. She was the youngest of four children. Her father Adolf had been married to Ella Strauss, a beautiful young woman from a wealthy family, who had died of pneumonia after going to a ball in the winter wearing a flimsy gown and catching a cold. Adolf was left with two young children, a boy called *Feri* (Frank) who was four and a girl called *Sarah* who was six years old. He needed someone to look after the children. It was customary in those days to be introduced through a marriage broker or a friend and one day soon afterwards he was introduced to the twenty eight year old Sarolta who was an intelligent, good looking woman. Adolf and Sarolta fell in love and married soon after their meeting. Their marriage was very happy. Two more children were born, a boy called *Imre* and two years later my mother *Miriam.* She was a beautiful child with big brown eyes and a charming round face and was also very bright but she only completed the eight years of compulsory education, leaving school at fourteen while her brother finished grammar school when he was eighteen. She picked up Latin grammar and vocabulary from his books and they both studied German, French and English probably from their mother and also had piano lessons. Miri was very good at sight reading and played the piano to a high standard. She was very fond of Chopin waltzes and Schubert songs but her brother Imre, who was more talented, hated practicing and had to be forced to sit at the piano. After leaving school Miri had ambitions to become an actress and had started studying at the Mattyasovsky-Bolváry Cinema School opposite their flat as *Vajda Mara*, but left after one year. Her report in May 1923 showed that she had achieved an excellent standard in voice production, dance and mimics, gymnastics and fencing as well as psychology and film acting. It is possible that by then the family fell on hard times and money was short for the second year. She very much admired the film star Lilian Gish and she had a certain resemblance to her idol. These were the early days of cinema, when films were silent.

There was a great deal of unemployment and hardship after the end of the First World War. Laws were introduced restricting the commercial activities of Jews. As a result many people emigrated to the United States or to Canada. The *Vajda* family (pronounced Voida) considered moving to Paris, so they first sent their son Imre at the age of eighteen or nineteen to find work and get established, and three years later when he started sending money home, Miri followed in the autumn of 1924 at the age of only 20. It is amazing to consider that her parents not only allowed but encouraged her to go and live in that far away big city at such a young age, but they were sure of her character and they trusted her completely. In Paris Imre changed his name to the more French sounding Raoul and Miri changed her name to Mimi after the heroine of La Bohéme by Puccini and this name stuck with her for the rest of her life.

She went to live with her brother on the sixth floor of 24 rue Beaurepaire, near the Place de la Republique. This is a large square with several roads leading from it which she found rather confusing, so Raoul told her to look in the direction in which the statue at the centre of the square was pointing with one arm lifted high to find her way home. There was no lift to the flat, it had a kitchen but no bathroom and a living room with only one bed which they had to share but she was very happy. The Swiss landlady objected to this arrangement saying that anyone can claim they are living with their sister. So Raoul had to move out into a hotel which cost him 8 francs a night.

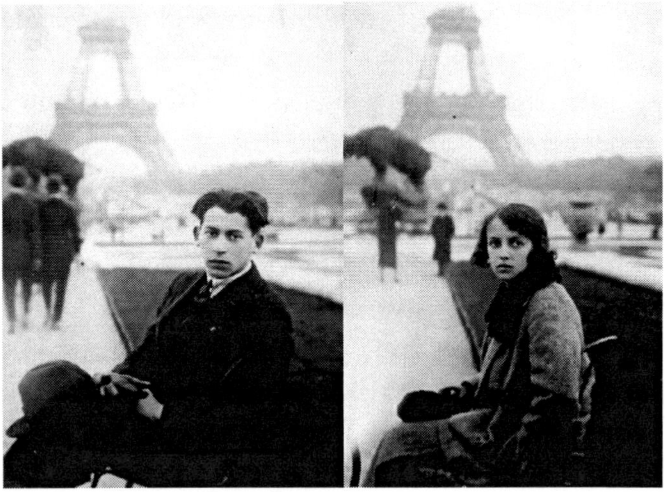

Raoul and Mimi on the 25th November 1924

There was an elderly seamstress next door called Mme Desgrange. Mimi spent many days sitting on a low stool helping her to thread needles and listening to her stories. She soon earned the title of '*Enfileuse d'aguilles*', or 'Needle Threader'. In the mornings her neighbour Mme de Vildreux came in with a cup of coffee for her friend. One day she invited Mimi to look inside her flat. There was a door to the kitchen another to the bathroom and the third to a living room and a bedroom. There was also a small room with a bed and Mimi asked her who slept there. Mme de Vildreux said it was her daughter's before she got married. So Mimi asked if she could move in there, but Mme de Vildreux had never let the room to anyone. So the next day Mimi asked their mutual friend Mme Desgrange to put in a word for her so that her brother could come back into his room from the hotel and she finally agreed. Madame de Vildreux became a very good friend and almost like a mother to Mimi. She was very kind to her and often invited her to share some of her homemade soup when Mimi returned home in the evenings after searching for a job. Mme de Vildreux asked what skills she had to offer, for example could she make hats and Mimi said, 'Yes, I did a course on hat making in Budapest.' So she suggested that Mimi should find a job as a milliner.

First she looked for a job on the Place Vendome and the Rue de la Paix where the best shops were found and one day she saw a notice on the shop window 'English speaking saleswoman wanted,' so she went in and when the owner asked 'Do you know how to make hats?' She replied 'Yes!' confidently. When there were no customers buying hats she was asked to work in the workshop. They gave her a hat to work on but she had no idea what to do! All the other girls were very accomplished, very good at their job, making beautiful hats and she watched their work with interest. At the end of the day the owner of the shop said, 'I am sorry we cannot employ you, but here is your day's salary'. So she went home to Madame de Vildreux who said 'Never mind, tomorrow you can find another place.' The next day she went into another shop in the Place Vendome and when she was offered the job told them 'I can only start next Monday'. Then into another shop she said 'I could only start next Tuesday' and so on. Eventually she had a job for every day of the week! Each day she worked in a different shop. Slowly she picked up enough knowledge and became quite good at millinery. But one day there were no more shops in the Place Vendome or the Rue de la Paix for a milliner. So Mimi had to go to the second best shops. She knew she was not good enough for the very best ones.

There was a workshop where they only made black hats for widows. She presented herself there, was offered the job and stayed for quite a long time, as they were satisfied with the quality of her work. There was a young man, the brother of the owner, who kept coming into the workshop, his name was Mark. Mimi heard that he was divorced and had a child. Later he proposed marriage to her, freely admitting that he needed someone to look after his child, but he also said he was in love with her. But Mimi did not want to marry anyone! Then he threatened her that he would join the Foreign Legion if she rejected him! She wondered how to deal with him so she told her brother about this young man who was pestering her to marry him and he forbade her to go back to the workshop. She went back with her brother in the morning to give in her notice and to collect her things.

Mark cried and pleaded with her on his knees not to go, he even went down to talk to her brother, but it was no use because Raoul's mind was made up.

Mimi had to find another job. She worked for a short time at the workshop of the Follies Bergère making huge props out of wire, which were covered with feathers, flowers and silks. The beautiful scantily clad ladies had to hold these on their heads with one of their hands and hold another as a fan as they danced on the stage. In another shop she made small handbags.

Mimi had a boyfriend called *Elbert Pista* who was a good looking, blond Hungarian boy. She had met him in Budapest during a ball at the *Aponyi Albert Polyclinic*, where she was one of the opening dance couples with *Dr Székely Lászlό*, who lived in the same building as her family. She had a lovely dress with flowers and beautiful high heeled shoes. *Elbert Pista* asked her to dance and he danced with her for the rest of the night. Later she met him again in Paris and he became very serious, wanting to get married, but she did not love him. He often came to visit and sometimes he was even waiting for her when she came home from work.

Mimi also had a Hungarian friend, called *Kondor Klári* who was a very flighty girl. One day a letter arrived saying that some friends had arrived from Budapest, *Glück Sanyi* and *Glück Ibi.* So they went to find them in the hotel where they were staying, but they were not in. There were three young men in the lobby; one from Argentina, one from England and the other from Holland. They started talking and the boys wanted to meet up again later that day. So the two girls agreed on a meeting place. But as

Mimi arrived home with her friend *Klári* she found *Elbert Pista* waiting outside anxiously. They did not want to tell him about meeting the three boys, so they made up a story about having to visit an old lady and he accompanied them to the bus stop. They got on the bus, but got off at the next stop and then walked back to the place where they were to meet the three boys. As they were walking towards the river Seine, Mimi in front with the Argentinean who was very keen on her, Klári behind with the other two boys, she turned back to see Klári gesticulating and saying that she was in great trouble! Then she saw Elbert Pista, who came by and he looked so astonished to see that she was walking with a stranger that he ran off! He realised that they told him a lie! He never came back after that.

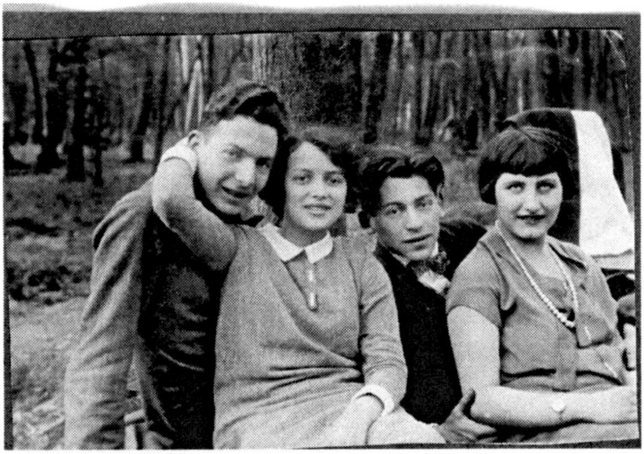

Mimi and Raoul in the centre with friends on a picnic.

Following this incident they met the three young men many times. Once when they went for dinner with them, Mimi made a drawing of the English boy, who was called George, on the white paper that was placed under the plate. Afterwards they went to the cinema, George was sitting next to her holding the picture she had drawn of him and he was crying. He had asked if she would wait for three years until he came back from working in a bank in British Columbia, but she said that she could not, because they did not know each other well enough. That was why he was crying.

My mother then answered an advertisement asking for someone to look after two boys who were four and six years old. She was interviewed by Mme Chouchon who hired her as a nanny and the next day she moved in with the family. She had to feed and dress the boys and take them for walks in a specially built large pram to the nearby park. The older boy had braces on his legs and one day he upset the pram up and fell out. Luckily he was not seriously hurt. The family owned a furniture shop on the Boulevard Magenta and had a young housekeeper.

Later she became a maid to an American lady called Mrs Jane Fuller, a sculptress, whose husband was an architect. In this position she was able to use her knowledge of English and the family took her on holiday to the South East coast of France to Saint-Jean-de-Luz. She often told me about this family and her experiences while she was working there. Mrs Fuller had a baby girl who was looked after by Mary, an American nanny, who was a Catholic. When she went on a visit to nearby Lourdes, my mother was left to look after the child, called Sage. She was a lovely little baby and although she was only two months old, Mary said she had to be held on a potty! But my mother had never seen such a young child held on a potty and she thought it was a very strange thing to do.

Mimi used to go swimming in the sea in the mornings before breakfast. At first the family watched to make sure that she was a good enough swimmer to be allowed to swim unsupervised. They were very caring and considerate. She was given a room in the villa right next to Mr. Fuller's room. One evening, quite late at night the chambermaid came to say that her cousin had arrived. She thought it must be her cousin Paul Biro who was also living in Paris! So she went down to meet him in her beautiful grey brocade dressing gown lined with red georgette, given to her by Mrs Fuller, but instead of her cousin she saw a stranger. She was very confused and went back to Mrs Fuller who was already in bed with her husband, and said 'There is a man here, who claims to be my cousin but I have no idea who he is.' Mrs Fuller got up straight away and went down and said to the man 'You get out of here, this is my house!'

She found out later that this man was a neighbour who came to the house to have drinks with Mr. Fuller, who told him, that there was a pretty young girl in their house and if he liked, he would introduce him to her. Mr Fuller was drunk when he went to bed but the neighbour stayed behind and then asked my mother to be called down.

When the Fullers went back to America they offered to take her with them but she decided to return to Paris. Later Mrs Fuller divorced her husband and married a publisher Cass Canfield and she kept in touch with my mother by correspondence. My mother took me to visit her when she was staying in London in 1958 and she gave me a watch. Their letters continued until she died in

1996. They were very fond of each other.

After she had been in Paris for three years Mimi's parents started sending letters asking her to go home to Budapest because her father was ill and they needed her to support them. She did support them from Paris sending most of the money she earned to them. She did not buy very much for herself. She told me that there were a pair of shoes she wanted very badly and she kept looking at them every morning for a long time before she eventually had saved enough to buy them. However she could not refuse her parents and decided to return to Budapest to help them. She said good bye to her friends and Raoul at the Gare de l'Est and set off on the long train journey. It took about fourteen hours. Her mother was waiting for her at the railway station in Budapest. When they arrived at the flat her father was leaning on the iron railing waiting for them looking very frail and unwell.

Mimi's mother said 'We live here like Les Miserables in Victor Hugo's novel', but they did not complain. They asked for an exchange so that they could move out of their previous flat on the first floor of Rákoczi út 24 where there was no lift and her father with his heart condition could not manage the stairs. They wanted a ground floor flat but instead were given a dreadful place. There were cockroaches crawling on the wall and they could not stay there. The neighbours asked Mimi's mother 'What does your daughter think of this place?' and her mother replied, 'She is so happy, she is singing all day like a little bird!'

On returning from Paris in 1928 Mimi went to see

the director of a large firm called NASICI, Dr Bártos Armin, whom she knew, to ask him if she could work there. There was a depression in Hungary and jobs were very difficult to find.

He said, 'You've come at a very good time Miriam! We have just started a parquet floor laying company on the first floor of this building, and they need a secretary.'

Mimi managed to get a very good, well paid job and as well as supporting her parents she could buy some carpets and the white bedroom furniture with raised decorations, her parents promised she could have if she came home from Paris. (The same white bedroom furniture stood in my bedroom when I was a little girl and we lived on the sixth floor). Although it was good job, her boss was not a good man. He cheated on his wife and had many affairs.

Mimi had to find another flat for her parents. Someone told her of some holiday homes outside Budapest in *Rákoshegy* where a family living there rented out a room because they needed the money. They had two daughters *Rolla* who was a doctor and *Ilona.* While they were staying there, Mimi was awakened one night by loud music outside. She looked out and saw a group of young men serenading, one was singing others playing instruments. The two girls looked out too, but the music was not for them. They were serenading Mimi! The young man singing was called *Dürner Laci*, who had fallen in love with her. Afterwards he often took her out on his motorbike; she sat on the pillion as they raced the trains going through the countryside. He was a quiet, unassuming young man who did not talk much.

Sometimes they stopped for a drink and he had a glass of beer but he never even tried to kiss her. This went on for months, until one day he stopped coming, nobody knew why.

After that summer she managed to find a ground floor flat in *Rákoczi út 61*. This was the same building where my father later moved in with his family on the first floor. Raoul had a friend *Frisch Tony* who also came home to Budapest from Paris. His mother was an upholsterer and Mimi often visited them to chat about life in Paris. Tony was very keen on table tennis and he took her to the Hungarian Tennis Club to play the game. He was a much better player than Mimi. At the club she met the slightly balding, very wealthy *Geiszt Gáspár*, known as *Gazsi* who was helping the club financially. He was a charming, well educated man and Mimi fell in love with him. There were some excellent tennis and table tennis players at the club. During the World Championships a group of English players arrived including Fred Perry. Mimi was paired with a man called Cyril Mossford from Cardiff. He had ginger hair and his father was an undertaker. They corresponded for a while after he returned to England but there was no talk of any romance. Mimi was not in love with him and they did not talk about anything personal because she was in love with *Gazsi*. She liked him very much although he was a very spoilt man who was used to having plenty of money and luxuries. He had a large property in the country at Csako and he often had to go there on business. He lived with his mother in a large villa on the *Andrássy út*, which is a very wide tree lined avenue with many expensive villas. It is one of the main avenues in Pest leading up to *Hősök Tere* (Heroes' Square). He even had a butler and when Mimi visited them, she realised that he would never marry her or anyone else. There was no future in their relationship, so although she was in love with him, she told him that she would never be his mistress because she was too proud and could not live with the prospect that one day he might say to her 'It was nice knowing you, now it is all over!' So they parted and he went on his way.

Soon afterwards my father Emil was passing in front of Adolf's front door with a radio in his hand and Adolf wanted to know what he was carrying. Emil told him that it was a radio that he had made and that he was an amateur radio enthusiast. This was in the early days of the development of radio. Emil also seemed to know quite a lot about electricity as he was a student at the Technical University. This must have been in 1930. My grandfather asked him to come and look at the faulty light fitting in the toilet and one day when Mimi returned from work he was working on it. That was how they met, in the toilet. Not the most romantic places to meet!

Emil had noticed her some time ago and admired her as she crossed the courtyard either in the mornings on her way to work or coming home in her big red coat.

Chapter 5.

Emil.

My father Emil was born in November 1910 in a tiny village called *Répceszentgyörgy* in the western part of Hungary where his father was the estate manager for the bishop of *Szombathely.* He was born just ten months after my grandfather *Bozzay Boldizsár* had married the seventeen year old *Horváth Margit.* A year and a half later another son *Dezső* was born who was nicknamed *Cincó* (pronounced Tsintso) by my father, imitating the sound made by a little mouse. This son, the naughty, mischievous one was my grandfather's favourite while my grandmother favoured Emil who was always more than happy to please her. They lived in a large house with servants and had a very good standard of living. *Boldizsár,* (Hungarian form of Balthazar) or Bodi for short, was a good looking, twenty eight year old young man, but slightly built and not very tall, who came from an old Hungarian noble family which could trace its roots back to 1271. They were the proud possessors of a family crest passed down through the eldest son. Margit was courted and won over by him and she decided to get married so that she could have her own household, be able to buy beautiful clothes and live a life of luxury with her own servants. Her father, Antal was also an estate manager from minor nobility with a good family background and her mother was a highly intelligent, well educated daughter of a doctor. Margit's three elder brothers were all teachers, the two oldest were educated in a seminary and the third József at an Art College. He became a famous, prize winning painter of aquarelles and the youngest son *László* followed in his father's footsteps by becoming a highly qualified, agriculturalist well known on television. The three girls in the family on the other hand were not educated beyond the compulsory six classes of primary school and a year or two at a finishing school. As girls were to be married it seemed a waste of money to educate them, but Margit was an avid reader and she decided to educate herself. As she was the eldest daughter in a family of seven children she was expected to contribute to the running of the household as soon as she was old enough. She married to escape these duties, believing that she was in love with Bodi. But the marriage was unhappy because she did not really love him. Margit was an outspoken, determined young woman who did not tolerate her husband's drinking, violent behaviour and subsequent loss of jobs. When the First World War broke out, many young men but not Bodi, went to fight and finding workers in agriculture was difficult. They had to move several times, finally ending up in *Szombathely* where Bodi's father was a high ranking official. Bodi tried to start a business but he was not successful. Margit had her first book of poems published and after twelve unhappy years of marriage left her husband. This was a very unusual step in those times and her family strongly disapproved of her decision. She had no support from them when she tried to start a new life in Budapest. First she worked as a seamstress and hardly earned enough to feed herself. Later she succeeded in becoming a journalist at the *Pesti Napló,* a popular daily paper, under the protection and guidance of the paper's editor *Lándor Tivadar.* He was a highly educated man who edited and encouraged her writing. After she had found a flat, Emil came to live with her. He was the responsible, sensible, reliable eldest child who grew up to be an athletic young man with the wide shoulders of a good swimmer. He was also very good looking with dark slightly curly hair and beautiful blue eyes. He had many admirers and girlfriends. His mother had high hopes for him as he was an able student and popular with teachers and fellow students alike. She planned a glittering future for him and probably hoped that she might have some returns for the large sacrifices she had made for his education, when finally he started to earn. She was planning to live in a villa with a garden together with her sons and possibly later, also their wives.

After leaving the *Vörösmarty Mihály* technical school in 1929 with excellent results Emil spent a year as a volunteer officer in the army. Conscription was compulsory but he had a privileged officer status as a volunteer member of the 'nobility'.

One of the highlight of his officer year was being the captain of the guards of honour at a glittering reception held for the Regent Horthy Miklós at the *Vigadó.* Emil was dressed in the period costume of Maria Teresia hussars, wearing a red chacko with white plumes over his white wig and an elaborately corded hussar jacket called an attila on his shoulder. After he finished his duties he danced with his mother at the ball. At thirty six she was exactly twice his age but they looked like a couple in love. She was very proud of her son's good looks.

The following September in 1930, Emil started his studies in Mechanical and Chemical Engineering at the *József Nádor* Technical University of Budapest, but he did not finish his studies. Maybe the course was too demanding, maybe mechanical and Chemical Engineering was the wrong course for him. He enjoyed technical drawing and was interested in science, but he was much more interested in the newly developing science of radio transmission. While he was at university he constructed and sold radios. He was also the editor of a radio journal called Antenna and later worked in the Remix laboratory that made radios. His mother was very unhappy about this as she had to make huge sacrifices to pay for his university tuition. It was a large expense for her even though she had a fairly good income as a journalist and writer.

Unfortunately Adolf died in the winter of 1931 and this was when Emil offered his condolences to my mother Mimi. This was the start of their serious relationship. They probably got engaged in November 1932, as this date is inscribed in her ring, but nearly three more years passed before the wedding took place in May 1935. By then the families had moved to different flats, Mimi and her mother lived in *Benzur utca* and Margit a short distance away in *Bajza utca 8*.

Emil did not finish his university studies to the disappointment and annoyance of his mother, instead he started working for Mimi's uncle William Biró whom she called *Vili bácsi* (uncle Vili). He was a wealthy industrialist with an engineering degree from Germany manufacturing fire extinguishing equipment and he changed his name from Rechnitzer to a more Hungarian sounding Biró. He later found Emil a better position in the offices of a large manufacturing firm making hunting rifles and ammunition.

Emil and Mimi were in love and wanted to get married even though both their mothers disapproved, but by the time Emil was twenty four he did not need parental consent according to the laws at that time.

Lotti wanted her daughter to marry a well established older man and arranged several introductions which were not welcomed by Mimi. Margit objected to the marriage because she wanted her son to finish his studies and not waste his life by marrying a poor Jewish girl who was six years older with neither an inheritance nor an aristocratic background, but came from a family of 'shopkeepers'. The Bozzay family was an ancient Catholic noble family with a family crest and she felt that her own background was similarly prestigious. She seemed to think so highly of the Bozzay name that she kept it even after she got divorced. To be a member of the nobility in Hungary had a certain prestige. Members of the nobility felt that they were better and more worthy than the 'peasant' class. They had to keep up certain standards of dress and behaviour and the education of sons was paramount. All five sons in the Bozzay family including my grandfather, who was the youngest, were university educated to become teachers, lawyers, or agriculturalists.

In spite of all this opposition Mimi and Emil decided to get married in secret in a registry office on Sunday the

12th May 1935 after three years of engagement. On this day my grandmother Lotti travelled to *Szombathely* on the train with her younger sister Riza, to tend the grave of their parents.

Strangely both my mother's and my father's families came from this ancient city near the Austrian border, one of the oldest cities in Hungary, which was established by the Romans as *Savaria*. Both my great grandmothers lived in the centre of the city, quite near each other at about the same time and both died aged forty nine, one in November 1892 and the other in November 1895. I sometimes wonder if they knew each other, maybe by sight and if they ever exchanged words when shopping in the market place. One was Jewish and the other a Catholic.

While their mothers were away, Riza's daughter *Marica* accompanied my parents to the registry office but they soon realised that a second witness was needed, so Mimi went out and stopped a passing stranger on the street to ask him to stand in and help them out. Afterwards they celebrated in a very beautiful coffee house called the *Lukács Cukrászda* on the *Andrássy út* the widest avenue in the city. When Mimi's mother returned home from *Szombathely* she was shocked to find that Emil was planning to spend the night there with her daughter but her objection melted away when he proudly pulled out the marriage certificate from his pocket and she realised that they were now legally married. I am not sure that she was pleased about the marriage taking place without her knowledge and against her advice, especially as Emil had few prospects and the newly married couple had nowhere to live except with her.

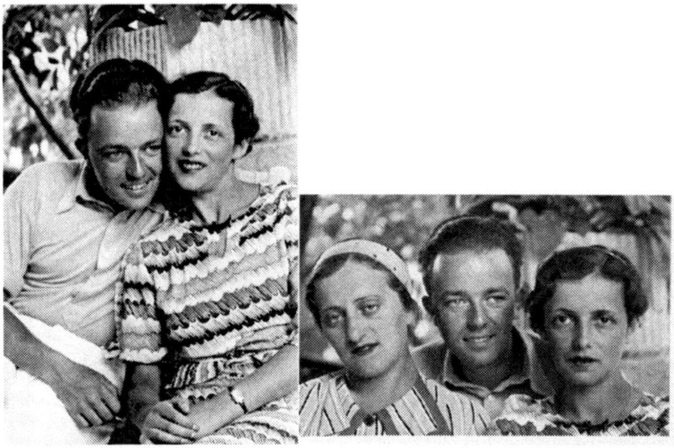

Marica, Emil and Mimi in May 1935.

For a few weeks Emil did not dare to admit to his mother that they had married. When he did she was devastated. He had asked her permission to marry my mother three years previously and when he was firmly refused, he promised to finish university and not to go against her wishes; but he broke his promise which hurt his mother deeply. They were very close, possibly because Margit was living on her own without the support of a man in her life. She felt betrayed and told him that she would never see him again, the worst punishment for a devoted son. She kept up this punishment for some time, but gradually relented. Even so, according to my mother, she tried to encourage the breakup of the marriage and possibly because of this she did not see me until I was three months old at Christmas. Although we lived only a few doors away from her in *Bajza utca* 2, she did not come to visit us, so finally my mother decided to take me to see her. She must have been won over by the sight of her first grandchild and the rift between the families was healed.

Unfortunately soon after this, in January 1942 she was diagnosed with ovarian cancer. Her stomach started to swell and she was beside herself with pain and worry. It was my mother who found a hospital bed for her and arranged for her admission and so earned herself a special place in Margit's affection. She was the only one who was allowed do her hair and makeup before visitors could see her. There was no hope of a cure, the cancer was too advanced. She wrote her last will in February, dividing her library of books between her sons, leaving her flat to her younger son Cincó and placed him into the care of her maid Böske. She left her silver cutlery to me, her only granddaughter and an amethyst dress ring to Mimi. She died on the 19th March 1942.

The funeral was a grand affair. She was a well known and much loved writer with many admirers. Four black plumed horses pulled the ornate black carriage piled high with tributes to the Kerepesi Cemetery followed by her contrite ex-husband, her faithful maid, her tearful sons, my mother and hundreds of fans. Her grave is in the best part of the cemetery where many famous poets and writers are buried and she has now been joined by her younger son, who became a well known industrial designer and his wife. A new marble memorial stone replaced the original wooden cross with an open book on which the final words of her last book, 'The Lesson Ends' are written, 'I have finished the task...I await your judgement'.

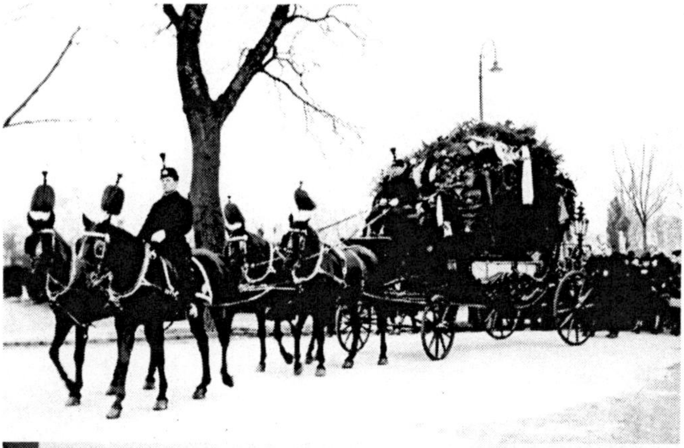

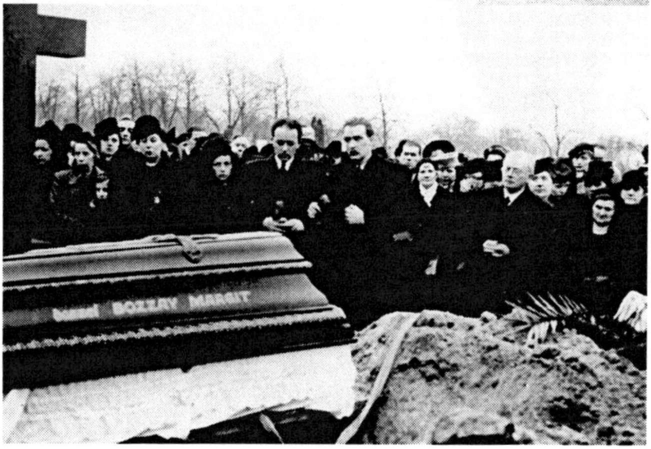

My mother and father, Cinco, my grandfather (with glasses) and Böske.

Chapter 6.

War years.

At the hospital where I was born on the 11th September 1941 the consultant was Dr Semmelweis, the great grandson of the famous Hungarian doctor Ignaz Semmelweis, who in the 1840s discovered that puerperal fever was caused by the failure of doctors, to wash their hands before examining pregnant women, after doing autopsies. That was how the infection spread to the women.

My mother often told me the story that as she was in labour in hospital, the doctor in attendance sat near her calmly reading a newspaper. He had nothing to do but wait for the imminent birth. My father and anxious grandmother waited outside in the corridor but as they could not hear any screams or noises my grandmother concluded that her daughter must be dead. I was born quite easily without any complications, the first and only child to my thirty seven year old mother.

If by telling me this story my mother was trying to impress on me that giving birth was not a frightening or an unbearably painful experience, she had certainly succeeded. I was well prepared for labour when I had my first daughter and had no difficulties giving birth; although even at twenty eight I was called an 'elderly prima gravida'. I had another daughter two years later who was born even more easily and our third daughter was born in the car on the way to the hospital eight years later when I was thirty eight. Maybe I was very lucky, but I believe that being frightened often increases the pain of childbirth.

Thirty seven was considered quite old to have a first child in 1941, although nowadays more and more women have their first child later in life. My parents had been married for six years already and I am not quite sure why they had waited so long. Maybe they were short of money and both salaries were needed, or maybe my mother had difficulty in conceiving.

My mother told me that she was trying to conceive for some time and when she did not succeed she went to see a gynaecologist who told her that she had an 'infantile womb'. I have no idea if there is such a condition and whether this was a valid explanation. She started to pray to St Anthony for help to conceive, as she had a great devotion to him. Three years before I was born she was baptised into the Catholic Church and she was very devout. Her prayers were answered and later when she met the gynaecologist as she was pushing me in a pram he was very surprised.

My mother also said that she wanted a child very much but my father was not so keen on the idea. There are many men who are reluctant to take on the responsibilities of a child and are not very fond of babies. My mother had to work hard to convince him. She told me that she even threatened him that if he refused her wish, she would ask the first stranger on the street, but I am quite sure that she would not have carried out this threat. She was probably feeling the effects of her biological clock ticking at thirty six while my father was still a young thirty year old. After I was born he became a loving, devoted, patient father and as he did not have a son, he often called me his daughter and son in the same person. He used to involve me when he was doing repairs or making things, taught me the names of his tools which I had to hand to him and called me his 'little apprentice.' He never refused to answer my questions and encouraged me in every way to do my best.

He was also keen to make me brave by standing me on top of the book case, which was about five foot six high and asking me to jump into his arms. Another favourite game was propelling me with his feet into a pile of cushions about eight feet away on the long divan made by linking their two single beds together at the short sides. My mother looked on anxiously in case he shot me off to the side, landing me on the floor but this never happened. He told me that I should never be afraid of anyone or anything. When I was about three we were in the attic and I tripped and fell against the corner of a piece of marble which made a deep cut above my eye. Blood was pouring down my face and my father carried me down to the bathroom to wash the wound. I was very frightened and cried 'Don't let me die!' He reassured me calmly and made me feel safe. Instead of being frightened of storms he taught me to work out the distance to the storm by counting the seconds between the lightning and the sound of the thunder.

For my bedtime reading my father found a book on astronomy by James Jeans called The Stars in Their Courses, published in 1931 and translated into Hungarian in 1942 as the Secrets of the Starry Sky and I was so entranced by the enormous size of the Universe, and the stories about the planets of the Solar System that for a long time my ambition was to study astronomy.

One of my earliest memories when I was about two and a half years old, is of the warm summer days spent in a small country village called *Csapdi*, about twenty miles east of Budapest. I was a treasured only child who arrived late in my mother's life and she was very proud of my looks. I had golden curls and blue eyes; my mother said that she drew several portraits of me before I was born, as if she were trying to design the child she wanted.

My father's best friend from his school days was *Olasz Ferenc*. He was always called *Franci* and his parents lived in this village. His wife *Lonci* was staying with them. She was a good friend to my mother and their daughter Eva was about my age. Our two mothers often took us on long walks through the woods and fields. At the time I did not realise that in fact my mother and I were hiding from the Germans who were deporting thousands of Jews mostly from the capital to the concentration camps. Jews had to wear a yellow Star of David, but my mother ignored the ruling. Although she had converted to Catholicism three years before I was born, she was still considered a Jew. Even I could have been deported by the Nazis, as I had two Jewish grandparents. My mother was a very resourceful woman, determined to survive, but many members of her family whether they put on the yellow star or not, disappeared, together with five hundred thousand Hungarian Jews.

Mimi was looking after the personal property of some Jewish friends which was a punishable offence at that time and some people in the small village of *Csapdi* became suspicious of her. Someone reported to the police that there were large suitcases in the house of the *Olasz* family which belonged to my mother. A policeman came and asked her to open the large chests which were kept at *Lonci*'s in-laws. But my mother had no idea which one of the many keys would open which chest. While she walked the small distance home to fetch the bunch of keys she prayed hard for help. By the time she returned, *Lonci* had charmed the policeman and he was in a much more favourable mood. To my mother's amazement the first key she tried, opened the first chest and she managed to convince the policeman that the contents all belonged to her. The police apologised and left, to her great relief.

June 6th 1944 was a memorable day for many reasons. In England it was the D-day landing when thousands of British and American soldiers were killed trying to land on the beaches of Normandy and my English cousin Stephen was born. His father Raoul was in the medical corps of the British Army. In Hungary the blue sunny sky was filled with planes and bombs were heard exploding in the distance. My parents in Csapdi were listening to the BBC World Service as usual, as it was the only reliable source of information and I went out in the sunshine to play next door. There was an old wine barrel collecting rainwater which stood at the corner of the neighbouring house with a seven foot drop next to it and there was no railing. The building had not yet been completed. Like all children I loved playing with water. I was pretending to be a washerwoman. At that time it was my greatest ambition in life to become one.

So when my mother called to me to come in for my afternoon sleep, I pleaded to be allowed to stay out for a few minutes longer. Suddenly I lost my footing and I was falling, falling... It was a wonderful sensation, I was flying through the air and I felt like a bird! I was not at all frightened; I really enjoyed the experience and often relived it in my dreams afterwards. But sadly my flight did not last very long. I landed on a pile of boulders. Strangely I have no memory of the pain which I must have felt. The next thing I can remember was being carried in the arms of our neighbour. As I looked down I could see that there was a big hump on my right thigh.

My mother later told me that she felt she was going to faint when she saw me in the neighbour's arms, as she realised that my leg was broken. There was a glass of water on the table and she quickly poured it over her own head.

My father stabilised the leg with two wooden spoons, wrapping it with a wet towel to reduce the swelling. He laid me on the back seat of his small black car with some cushions and gave me my doll to hold for comfort. During the drive to Budapest to find a doctor, I dropped the doll several times and had to ask my mother to turn round and pick it up.

There was an air raid in Budapest. The houses were in ruins, the roads were almost impassable, but my father managed to find the professor, a family friend and drove him to the small clinic near our flat where with the help of his wife he put my leg in plaster. As she lifted my leg in the still soft plaster, she accidentally made a dent at the heel as she was not a trained nurse.

A few weeks later I started complaining, 'My leg hurts, my leg hurts!' But I couldn't explain where it was hurting. So my mother took me to the hospital in Esztergom, where we had recently moved, to be near my father's army unit. He had not yet been called up to fight on the Western front and was hoping that the war would end before that happened.

The doctor in the hospital could not understand the reason for the pain, so my leg was X-rayed and it was found that the professor had not joined the bones correctly. The bones were overlapping and if it was left like that my right leg would be shorter. When my mother returned home and explained to my father that my leg would have to be broken again and joined correctly under X-ray he was incredulous. He could not believe that an experienced professor could make such a mistake. But my mother assured him that she saw the X-ray and that there was no doubt about it.

She was determined and always had her way, and so it was decided that my right thigh bone would have to be broken again and I was taken into the operating theatre. When the plaster was taken off they discovered that there was a wound caused by the dent at the heel. This was why I was in so much pain and if the plaster had not been removed the wound would have turned to gangrene. I was very lucky not to have lost my foot or even my leg.

I remember clearly my father standing behind me, as I lay on the operating table, with his hands tightly clenching my temples and saying, 'You must be brave!' as two or three men got hold of my right leg and pulled it hard. There was probably excruciating pain, because it was not considered necessary, or maybe I was too young to be given anaesthetics. I almost certainly cried out, although I don't remember it. My mother outside in the corridor must have felt dreadfully anxious.

The leg was put into plaster again, this time under guidance of an X-ray machine and my leg was put in a pulley vertically in the hospital bed. When the plaster was removed I had to learn to walk again the second time in my life.

In October 1944 news came that the Russians were advancing and my parents wanted to return to Budapest, but they could not find a removal van until the beginning of November. The war was still being fiercely fought and during bombings people took shelter in the basement cellars of large blocks of flats. We stayed in such a cellar under the building where my grandmother Margit had lived, with about twenty other families. People put their beds or mattresses close together by the wall and someone found a stove which could be heated by coal. There was a large coal store behind a door in the corner which was used to fuel the central heating system for all the flats in the house. It was a spacious cellar, about seven feet high with dirty grey walls, tiny windows at the street end high up near the ceiling, concrete floors and several large square pillars supporting the ceiling. There were a few tables and chairs and people spent their time playing cards, chatting to friends or reading. They shared their food and my mother was happy to do the cooking for five or six families on the small stove in the centre of the cellar. Food was scarce, but she could make soup from dried vegetables. When there was a short lull in the bombing, people could go back into their flats to fetch supplies.

I had a friend in the cellar called *Jancsi* (John). We liked to pretend that we were married; playing mothers and fathers, so I called him my husband and he called me his wife. John had a small red pedal car which I thought was a wonderful toy and there was enough room to sit next to him as he pedalled round the pillars. We imagined that we were going on outings or holidays, as he pedalled round and round the big pillars of the cellar and we made the best of being stuck in a dark, dusty place.

One day as we were happily playing and my mother was preparing dinner, a stray bullet entered through one of the narrow windows. We were very frightened. There was a loud crack, people were shouting in terror as they were running for shelter. The bullet hit a rather large lady in her buttock. She cried out in pain as she fell to the floor and several men rushed to her aid. They lifted her up high and carried her off somewhere. I have no idea where she was taken. It seemed very amusing to us children and we laughed about it for a long time, but in retrospect it was not at all funny. I now feel very sorry for the poor woman who must have been in great pain.

One morning we were awakened by the heavy sounds of exploding bombs. It was the final battle for Budapest fought between the German and Russian armies. The sky was filled with planes. The German army blew up all the bridges across the Danube as they were retreating. Budapest was surrounded by Russian troops.

Later that day a Russian soldier came into the cellar. People greeted him joyfully; some of the women even kissed his rough face. One of the women who could speak Russian greeted him and asked his name. He said his name was called Sergei. The people in the cellar were glad to see him because they thought that he was bringing news of the end of the war.

'*Ora? Ora van*?' ('Watches? Any watches?') He called in his broken Hungarian.

As he collected watches from the willing donors they noticed that his arm was festooned with several watches right up his arm, but still he wanted more. My mother refused to hand over her watch, deciding to save it for some future occasion. Many of the Russian soldiers came from small villages and had never seen a wristwatch. They were fascinated with watches and often took them to pieces to find out what made them work. Later they discarded them as they could not put the pieces together again.

When the soldier saw me, he sat down and lifted me on his knee. I may have reminded him of his small daughter he had left behind. After a short time he said something to my mother and left. Later he came back with a bag of sugar for me, which was a very welcome gift in those days of food shortages.

Not all the Russian soldiers were kind. There was Nicolai, who was a captain, judging by his uniform. He came with a group of his men and asked for food. The people in the cellar gave them as much as they could find. As they were sitting round the table eating, a Hungarian woman who understood them realised that they were talking about girls. She alerted the other women and advised them to hide. But Nicolai had already set his eyes on the attractive fifteen year old girl who was being looked after by my parents. Her name was *Veronka* and she was an orphan from Esztergom. Her Jewish parents were taken away by the Nazis and probably died in the concentration camps. Nicolai decided to take *Veronka* into one of the more sheltered parts of the cellar behind the closed door where the coal was kept. We could hear her cries coming from there but no one dared to go to her aid. He came back a few days later brandishing a revolver and asking for *Veronka* again. It was impossible to hide the young girl from his unwanted attentions. After the war ended she went back to her home town and later took her own life.

It was during this winter that my grandmother Sarolta became ill and was in hospital about ten minutes from where we took shelter in the cellar. Sarolta was suffering from uterine cancer and there was no treatment. My mother visited her every day and took her food. Sometimes she had to run through the street while bombs were falling and explosions caused broken glass to fall about her. She was very brave and devoted to her mother. One day when she arrived she found her mother asleep and she bent over to kiss her. Then the patient in the next bed told her that her mother had died during the night. Mimi screamed out in pain, but there was no one to console her.

A coffin had to be found, so she went to the supplier and dragged it through the snow covered streets like a sledge all the way to the hospital. When she arrived she could not find her mother. They had put her body out into the courtyard together with several others. She was not strong enough to search for her, so she asked my grandfather to help. He found her body and it was placed in the coffin. She was buried in the far corner of the Kerepesi Cemetery unlike Margit whose grave was near the main avenue among the famous. The headstone over her grave was inscribed *Vajda Adolfné, Rechnitzer Sarolta 71 years old.*

German occupied Budapest was liberated by the Russian army on the 4th April 1945 but the euphoria of the people was short lived. Hungary became a Republic, democratic elections were held, and a coalition government was formed. But the Hungarian Communist Party, supported by the occupying Soviet army, did not accept the result of the democratic process. The elected government was overthrown by unlawful arrests, deportations to Siberia, and other violent means. The communists assumed power and introduced a reign of terror which resulted in the Hungarian Revolution of 1956 and lasted until 1989.

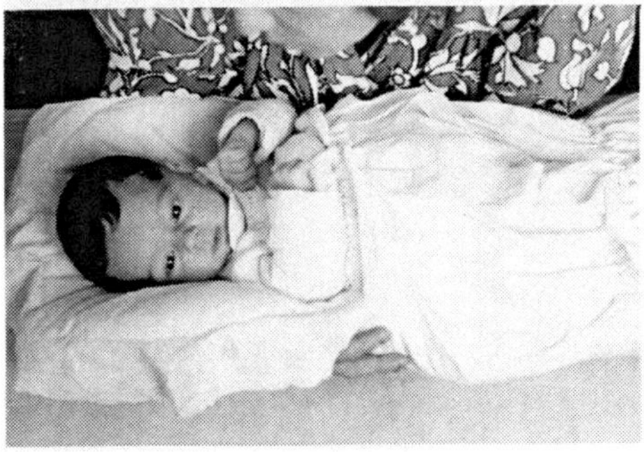

Zsuzsi in September 1941

Chapter 7.

Living with polio.

In the late autumn of 1949 when I was eight years old, after our failed attempt at escaping, I lay paralysed in an isolation ward with six or eight empty beds and windows overlooking the hospital gardens. The paralysis which started to affect my left side was progressing from my left foot up to my leg, then to my left arm and reached the left side of my face. I developed a strange lop sided smile.

I could not to sleep at night so my father paid for a nurse, who was also a nun, to sit next to my bed. All through the night I sang songs I had learnt at school, mostly communist ones. When my father came to visit me in the evenings after work I asked him to put his arm under the aching small of my back so as to lift it up from the bed. This gave a wonderful relief from the pain.

Four times a day a doctor visited me to administer a whole series of injections into the vein on the back of my hand, consisting of vitamins to boost the immune system and some blood from a woman who had had polio, in the hope that it contained some of her antibodies and it would be transferred to me to destroy the virus. The doctor joked as he gave me one injection after the other, saying that he came to give me dinner. The first one was the starter; the second was the main course and finally came the pudding. I did not complain, I knew that it was for my good, but soon the back of my hand started to look like a pincushion. I lay in the hospital bed unable to move and hoping that my mother would come soon.

To my great joy she was released from prison a week later and arrived at the hospital. We hugged each other and I was so relieved to have her by my side. She insisted on being given a bed next to mine and for the first time since I came into hospital I slept through the night.

The nurses at this hospital were nuns with large winged head dresses and they were very kind. They were Sisters of Mercy and the Reverend Mother had been praying hard to avert the paralysis from reaching my lungs. If it had affected my lungs I would have died because there were no iron lungs available. The only two iron lungs in the country were already occupied. Later she gave me a small Miraculous Medal to remind me that her prayers had been answered and she made me promise that I would wear it for the rest of my life.

I probably contracted the disease at the orphanage, because I was so exhausted and malnourished in those last few weeks before I had developed the symptoms. Polio hits those who are in poor health harder. I recently found out that out of a hundred people who are affected by the viral infection of poliomyelitis only one person ends up paralysed while most of the others are not even aware that they had polio. But many years later they might all suffer from Post Polio Syndrome with symptoms such as pain and weakness.

My mother must have been distraught to see me so ill and I sometimes wonder if she blamed herself for taking me on that long adventure to escape from communism. If she did I was never aware of it, neither did she show any distress about my condition. She accepted things as they were and was determined to rehabilitate me. Her acceptance helped me to cope with my illness and overcome my difficulties. I owe a great deal to her.

I stayed in hospital for about four weeks. It was nearly Christmas when we arrived home. In Hungary the main celebrations take place on Christmas Eve and in the afternoon I was carried off for a special bath. It was full of herbs floating on the warm water and smelt very nice but it looked a horrid brown colour. When I was finally carried back into our room there was a large Christmas tree lit up with coloured lights and covered with 'angel hair' which was in fact glass fibre. This has the magic effect of encircling the lights with coloured haloes. Under the tree were more presents than I had ever seen before. There were many books which were unwrapped standing up slightly open and a small children's prayer book with a beautiful picture of Mary and the baby Jesus on the hard shiny cover which I still treasure. Inside my mother inscribed "May God heal you, guard you and lead you on all your journeys."

My mother started a regime of daily exercises. I have no idea where she found the information for the method that she used. She must have spent much time in researching and finding out what she had to do to rehabilitate me. My left arm was paralysed so to encourage the return of muscle tone it was held in a strap above my head and tied to the headboard. This was not a very comfortable position but I did not complain. My mother had met another family with a teenage daughter who was also paralysed by polio. But when she recommended this procedure to them, the young girl refused to have her hand held in that position as she found it too uncomfortable. Possibly as a result of this her arm did not recover.

We started the exercises at nine in the morning, and continued after a short break for lunch. My mother sat by my bed until three in the afternoon lifting the floppy limbs one by one and encouraging me to hold them by myself. Gradually there was a flicker of movement which over the weeks grew stronger. I am sure I would not have been able to carry out all these exercises on my own. My mother had the determination and the vision to keep going. She was not going to give up. To stop me from getting bored she read stories to me. One of these was The Count of Monte Cristo by Alexandre Dumas which I enjoyed very much although it was not written for an eight year old child. It captured my imagination and after we had finished the book my mother found the sequel called The Son of Monte Cristo. She spent many months reading to me while doing the exercises to get me walking again. She had great perseverance.

Gradually the paralysis left me and my crooked smile disappeared. My left arm started to move and every day there were tiny improvements giving me hope and lifting our spirits. At first I could only get about on all fours, later I learned to walk leaning on the back of a chair using it like a zimmer frame to give me support. We had a small folding child's chair and our next door neighbour's three year old little girl copied me by leaning on this chair. Suddenly the chair folded up and her little finger was trapped. The top of her finger was sliced right off. The child screamed. My mother came into the room and calmly replaced the top of the finger. Then she and the child's mother took her to the hospital, but the cut was so fine that it was hardly visible at all. The doctor could not understand why they had come to the hospital! My mother always had presence of mind in a crisis.

Later I was given two crutches and with the help of these I took three steps unaided after one year. It was a special birthday present for my father on his 40th birthday, the 17th November 1950. It felt like a huge achievement and I was very proud of myself. This was the best present I could have given my father and he cried with joy. This was the third time in my life I had learnt to walk!

Somebody told my mother about the famous Pető Institute where paralysed children were rehabilitated and she decided to take me there for an assessment. The Institute had a very good reputation but it was difficult to be accepted for treatment. The great man was sitting in the centre of the room with several people around and examined me as I was sitting on the floor in front of him and said to my mother, 'If I stretch my thumb like this, all the muscles in my body start to work!' My mother just looked at him in disbelief, thinking that this man must be crazy. Later we were shown round the Institute and saw a large number of children sitting on the floor in another room singing Communist marching songs and waving their arms about. They could not stand or walk, so they exercised their arms instead.

After my examination the famous Pető said to my mother, 'Your daughter is accepted for treatment!' He went on to explain that I would have to be left at the

Institute and my parents would be allowed to visit me once a month. My mother was shocked at this news, thanked him and turned down the offer. She was not going to leave me there on my own for a month. The family and most of our friends thought that she had made a big mistake, but she was convinced that she had made the right choice.

I think Pető realised that I was a suitable candidate to enforce his image of being a great healer, because he could see that I had possibilities and would get better. That was why he was ready to take me. He was a staunch communist who was sponsored by the Communist Party. My mother took me to several other doctors, some of them advised that I should have an iron 'body belt' to stop my spine from getting a curvature, and others who recommended callipers. Thanks to my mother I did not have to put up with any of these horrible, uncomfortable 'aids' until very recently. She saw children in callipers with completely wasted limbs and concluded that if a muscle is not used it will atrophy.

The long hours of daily exercises brought the benefit of slow but sure recovery. I am very grateful to my mother for all she did for me because without her perseverance I would not have been able to achieve what I did. Our escape from Hungary had been unsuccessful but at least we were together as a family. We made the best of our life but my mother never gave up hope that one day we would be able to go to England and see her brother.

I lost two years of schooling due to my illness but my parents made sure that I was not left behind in my education. In Hungary every child has to pass an exam before being allowed to enter the next year. Near the end of the school year in 1951 my mother took me to school where I was allowed to take an aural exam in the summer and having passed it, was allowed to enter the next class. Unfortunately I was not very good at remembering dates, so when the teacher asked me the date of the liberation of Hungary, meaning at the end of the Second World War by the Soviet army, I answered '1954' instead of '1945' which caused loud laughter and shouts of 'If only it were true!' The year was 1951 and the teachers were hoping to be liberated 'from' the Russians. Even though I gave the wrong date I passed the small aural exam. I did not continue in the same school because we were soon to be moved to another flat in Buda on the other side of the Danube.

One night, before we had moved, we were all in bed, but not quite asleep, there was a loud knock on the door. My mother quickly put my father's gold watch into her shoes and went to open the door. There were two uniformed policemen with rifles demanding to be allowed in. They were checking for undesirables because there was a big party at the Romanian Embassy nearby. The family we were sharing the flat with had a visitor, who had arrived that evening and had not yet registered with the police. This was considered to be a crime and they took him away. He was never seen again. When they left, we saw the lights come on one by one in all houses across the road. The police were checking all the neighbouring houses for possible troublemakers.

Chapter 8.

Moving to Buda.

The authorities wanted the garden villa, where we lived, for a consulate and offered to re-house us in a first floor flat in Buda, opposite the Cog Railway. It was a spacious and modern flat with two large interconnecting rooms, two bedrooms, one quite large and the other tiny, a kitchen, a bathroom and a balcony. There were four doors in the entrance hall. On the right of the entrance was a door to the second toilet, next to it a door to the kitchen, straight ahead a door to a small room where Böske, my grandmother's maid lived until she passed away and the fourth on the left opened to the large living room. There were double glazed windows, with panes of glass that had a large enough space between them for a boot or a shoe that I hoped would be filled with sweets on the 6th December, St Nicholas' day if I was good. There was no chimney and no Father Christmas. The floor was covered with basket weave parquet and the central heating was supplied from boilers in the basement. There were two flats on each floor on each side of the lift and two more flats on each mezzanine floor. On the top floor just above the fourth floor there was a laundry room and a large rooftop with space to dry the washing or just to sunbathe. It was like a large balcony with a stone balustrade all around to make it safe.

We moved in and soon my parents managed to get back their furniture by paying off the storage fees. When it arrived I was amazed to see the old dining table that I used to play under. It seemed to me to have shrunk in storage, but of course I had grown! Everything fitted in well. The two beds in the bedroom were on either side of the bathroom door. The large unit with bureau, display shelf and wardrobe against the wall opposite the bathroom door with the glass topped round table in front of it with two armchairs on either side. There was also a record player and radio cabinet and my father made a large round lighting unit for the ceiling which contained the loudspeaker. He was very fond of classical music which blasted out at a very high volume. At the foot of one of the beds stood a plant stand with wrought iron legs, supporting two shelves with palms and other houseplants next to the door to a small balcony. In the living room near the window stood my grandmother's writing desk with her picture above next to the family crest, and my father's wardrobes were standing next to the desk. The book cases which were designed to stand next to the wardrobe were stacked on top of each other in an alcove on other side of the door with the telephone resting on its wall hung shelf. We also had a large settee covered with gold coloured velvet, inherited from my grandmother and the dining table with six chairs and the china cabinet which I believe were designed by my uncle *Cincó* who gave them to my parents in 1942. The large china cabinet had to stand in front of the second door to the bathroom, but one door from the bedroom was sufficient.

Another advantage of the move apart from the extra space was the excellent school nearby named after Lorántffy Zsuzsanna the wife of my hero from the eighteenth century, the leader of the uprising Prince Rákóczi Ferenc II. I was enrolled and started in the primary school for the next three years and then after passing the Small Matriculation exam, I progressed to the grammar school which was in the same building.

I walked very slowly at first, using two crutches for about a year, later I progressed to only one crutch to help my balance. My mother took my arm every morning as we made our way up the steep hill through derelict grounds destroyed by bombs during the war, next to our block of flats, and then up the steep hill to the school. I could not carry my school bag, so my mother met me at one o'clock when school ended.

Twice a week an energetic, lively physiotherapist called Mári néni, (Aunty Mary) came to our flat twice a week in the afternoon. She was probably in her sixties but she wore bright colourful dresses like a twenty year old, had short blond hair and walked with a spring in her step. She had been trained in the USA at the Sister Kenny Institute which was a famous place for people who had polio and she had achieved excellent results with her patients. I lay on the carpet doing the exercises and at the same time she taught me the Latin names of the muscles, pointing out their origin and insertion. She made me promise that I would carry on exercising every day for the rest of my life, which I promised to do but later neglected, except for short periods when I felt guilty. She was an excellent teacher and I started to make great improvements with her help.

My father's job improved when he was promoted to an executive position in '*Duclos*', (the company with the name of a famous French communist). They made mining machinery and in the mornings my father was picked up by a large black limousine. I was allowed a lift in this car to the school. The car waited outside the gates while my father helped me up into the main hall and he ran up the stairs to the first floor classroom with my school bag while I slowly followed. All the lessons were in the same class so my class mates and I did not have to move around, instead the teachers came to us. This must have made my mother's life a little easier as she had only to come and collect me from school at one o'clock.

We did not have much money for clothes; most of mine were made from second hand ones sent from America by my mother's Armenian friend Mina. They had met in Paris in the 1920s and she was now living in the US. I think she collected the clothes from her friends and acquaintances. The clothes first had to be unpicked then re-cut before being sewed up again. We had a dressmaker who came to the house to do this, but the unpicking was my job. Needless to say I hated it, nearly as much as I hated trying on the clothes and standing still to have the hems pinned up. Once she sent a dress which fitted me without any alterations, it was black with coloured fruits printed on it, had a full circle skirt and a fitted waistline. I loved this dress and I felt very grown up in it. I also loved a shiny jacket with a zip in the front which was bright green with bright yellow raglan sleeves, and was told that it was the kind that jockeys wear when racing.

In the spring, when the weather turned warmer, all the winter clothes were packed away in a suitcase and the summer clothes taken out. They seemed like new after being hidden for 6 months.

We made friends with the *Bozzai* family who lived on the fourth floor. They were possibly distant relatives as they almost shared our name. *Manci* was married to *Pista*, a butcher and their ten year old son was called *Pityu*, (both Pista and Pityu are diminutives of Stephen). One day my mother was making a collection for the caretaker, knocking on all the doors in the building. In large blocks of flats in Budapest there is always a caretaker who lives on the ground floor and looks after the building, such matters as the servicing of the lift, looking after the central heating boiler in the basement, cleaning the staircase and putting out the rubbish. When she knocked on *Manci*'s door on the fourth floor she found her in a desperate state. She wanted to jump out of the balcony because her husband was late coming home and she suspected that he was having an affair. My mother persuaded *Manci* to come down to us on the first floor where she would see him returning home. She said that he would be very worried when he found her gone and the fright would teach him a lesson. She also acted as their marriage guidance counsellor and sorted out their differences. The plan worked and we became very good friends with them. *Pista* was a handsome, charming man who used to bring us pork chops or other meat for the week end. In the days of shortages others had to queue for meat and were lucky if they managed to get any. As the friendship developed the four grown-ups started to play canasta, a card game which they enjoyed very much while *Pityu* and I got up to some mischief on the balcony. We used to drop small coins from there when it was getting dark and time the fall so that they landed just behind an unsuspecting pedestrian. Then we watched with great amusement as the person bent down looking on the pavement to find the money they thought they had lost. We also threw small pebbles on the roofs of passing buses which made a nice clanging sound and sent paper aeroplanes with lighted matches in their tails into the dark night.

'Aunty' Manci and *'Uncle' Pista* treated me like a daughter and I too was very fond of them. I felt sorry for their son who was younger than I because they hardly ever had a good word for him. They had an early cine camera and filmed the progress of my walking. We often went on picnics with them to the hills of Buda. One day while our parents were talking, Pityu and I started to climb the steep hill with its winding, zigzagging path. We avoided the paths and just climbed straight up. When my parents noticed our absence they started to look for us and asked people coming down the path if they saw us, but nobody did. They became very worried. When they eventually found us we were told off with stern words. My father slapped my leg, a punishment which I did not mind at all. I understood that he loved me and was very upset, but my mother never forgot it. She often reminded me of this incident and blamed my father for losing his temper with me.

In the winter we often took the Cog Railway to the top of the hill and found a long slope where we could slide down on our sledge. It was so cold that I had to have several layers of clothing to stop my feet from freezing. When 'Uncle Pista' bought a BMW motorbike he took me for a short ride on the main road. It was a great thrill to be sitting on the pillion seat and doing 100 km an hour! My mother waited for me anxiously by the gate hoping that I would be returned in one piece.

I never thought of myself as 'disabled'. There was nothing that I could not do; I just had to find a different way of doing it. As I was making progress all the time there was no reason to be despondent. My parents never showed that they were upset by my disability and they never implied that they felt sorry for me. Yet it must have been a terrible burden for them to see their only child so ill and incapacitated. I realise this now, having had children of my own. There is nothing worse for parents than seeing their children ill. But my parents were very positive and always gave me confidence. It was only when I saw myself walking towards a mirror that I realised that I did not walk like others. My self-image was always that of a normal person.

My friend Magdi and her family who used to live opposite us were deported to the country. Many families in Budapest lost their flats and all their belongings in the raids of 1952. Police arrived in the middle of the night and told people to pack what they could. They were then taken to a far away village and given a room in a peasant's house. They were not allowed to return to the capital and had to endure dreadful living conditions. Their flat in Budapest was confiscated and given to a communist party member. After some time Magdi and her family were allowed to come and visit us every week when they used our bath as there was no such thing where they lived. Afterwards we used to play Red Indians, making up Indian names for ourselves and trying to make a tepee. I read a book by a Hungarian man who became a Dacota Indian in the United States and this gave us ideas for making all kinds of Indian jewellery and dress.

On the morning of March 5th 1953 we woke up to the news on the radio that Stalin, the hated leader of the Russian Communist Party had died. He was a tyrant and a ruthless dictator who represented the occupying Russian forces in our country. Anyone who stood in his way was either executed or else sent to the Gulag in Siberia. He had promoted a benign picture of himself, like a favourite uncle, protector of little children but we knew that he was not to be trusted. Now Stalin was dead and all we could hear on the radio was the Funeral March by Chopin played over and over again all day long.

My mother took me to school as usual carrying my school bag and supporting my left arm while I walked with a crutch. When we arrived at my classroom we found that the teacher had not yet arrived. Instead of the teacher, one of my class mates, the daughter of a government minister and member of the communist party, was sitting on the podium. Her eyes were red from crying and she was holding a handkerchief as she was wiping her eyes. She had something to cry about because her family had many privileges, such as a big house, car and plenty of money. My mother and I were so happy, we could hardly contain ourselves, but we had to hide our joy. My mother almost burst out laughing and had to cover her face with her hand and quickly turn round before she left me in the class. That day was a memorable one for me, in some ways similar to the day Kennedy was shot. Everyone who was alive on that day remembers what they were doing when they heard the news.

The other hated figure was *Rákosi Mátyás*. He was born *Rosenfeld Mátyás*, the son of a Jewish grocer and he repudiated all religions including Judaism. Bald headed and fat, he was the General Secretary of the Communist Party and the dictator who ruled from 1945 to 1956 using the same methods as Stalin in Russia. He was trained in Moscow and he copied his teacher Stalin in every way. In fact he claimed to be 'Stalin's best pupil'. He was responsible for two thousand executions, a hundred thousand imprisonments and expelling two hundred thousand communists from the party for criticising his policies. His picture was prominent in all places next to those of Stalin and Lenin. Flowerbeds were created with the words "Long live Rákosi!" and on May 1st 'Workers' day' and on April 4th 'Liberation day' he stood under the oversized statue of Stalin saluting the army marching in front of him. It is not a very nice thing to admit but at school my friends and I were fantasising about how we could torture and kill Stalin and Rákosi.

All the children in the primary school had to be members of the Communist organisation called 'Young Pioneers' which was modelled on the scouts but without any religious content. There was no choice. We were given triangular red neckerchiefs to be worn with white blouses and had to swear allegiance to the Communist party. We were gathered together in the big hall of the school for the ceremony. But instead of saying our names we mumbled something so as to make the promise invalid. Apparently some of the children enjoyed summer camps with their fellow pioneers but I never joined any of the activities if I could help it! Later, people were forced to join other Communist organisations in order to get into University or get a job.

In the final year of primary education when I was thirteen, we had the opportunity to have dancing lessons and I joined in trying to learn the waltz to the best of my ability. I found it quite difficult. I was also offered music lessons on an instrument of my choice. I wanted to play the piano even though we did not have room in our flat for one. There was an aptitude test which I passed, as I was good at singing, recalling a tune and clapping a rhythm, but I was told that my hands were not suited to play the piano. I was advised to learn the 'cello, but I was a stubborn child and refused, so I had no music lessons.

I was not only stubborn but also a lazy child at school. I did not like doing my homework. Compulsory lessons in Russian started at the age of 11 and I hated this language because it was that of our oppressors. We made the poor Russian teacher's life a misery by throwing paper missiles, shouting and misbehaving in every possible way. At the end of the 8th year in June 1954 we ceremoniously burnt our Russian books in the middle of the road in front of the school! As a result of resisting the lessons, I know hardly any Russian, although I can still read the alphabet. I feel sorry now that I missed the opportunity to learn another language which might have been useful.

At that time there was the final examination called Little Matriculation in the main subjects, such as

Hungarian literature, Maths, History and General Science, but luckily not in Russian. There were about 100 questions in each subject and having memorised the answers, each person had to go into the examination room selecting one of these questions at random written on cards and placed face down on the desk. There were three examiners and while the previous person was giving the answers, the next candidate had 10 minutes or so to prepare their response to the question selected. The examiners could then ask further questions. It was similar to a 'viva'. This sort of test did not require much thought, only good recall and I passed quite easily. Those who did not pass would have gone to a vocational or technical school instead.

I was allowed to enter the first year of Grammar School which was to last four years. This was fortunately in the same building as the Elementary School. There was a school report in February and also at the end of the year which showed that I had made great improvements. I managed to gain top marks (5) in History, Latin, Chemistry, Geography and Singing, whereas before I had a 5 only in Singing. But I was quite poor in Russian, Hungarian language and literature, only getting a 3. As I had a very inspiring chemistry teacher, I learned to love the subject and I decided to become a chemist! My parents encouraged this ambition and my mother told me that she had a cousin, *George Biederman*, who was a professor of Chemistry in Stockholm.

In July 1955 I went to hospital to have my first operation. Both of my feet were floppy and I often tripped because I was not able to lift my toes. I had to wear lace up boots to hold the feet but I was longing to be able to wear fashionable shoes which at that time were 'ballet shoes'. The surgeon transplanted the tendon which lifts the big toe on the right foot to the instep and this helped to lift the whole foot. The operation was very painful because the Achilles tendon had to be lengthened at the same time by cutting a zig zag into it and then stretched before the foot was put into plaster. I hated the after affects of the ether anaesthetic. It made me feel nauseous for days afterwards. So when I was due to have the next operation in the summer of 1956 on the left foot, which had no working muscles at all and had to be fixed, I pleaded with the surgeon to let me stay awake!

I was given injections of a local anaesthetic and could watch the progress of the operation in the shiny central part of the overhead mirror. It was quite painful at times, and I could hear hammering and the cutting of tendons, but I did not mind as long as I avoided the dreaded ether. I was still hoping for the nice ballet shoes which I would be able to wear soon and the pain was worth it to achieve this. Sadly I was told after the operation that yes, I could wear them but really it would not be a good idea. So I had to carry on wearing the horrid lace up boots for many more years. The only concession was that I could choose the colour.

It was during one of these hospital stays that I met *Nyiredi Csaba* who also had polio and was going to have an operation on his shoulder by the same surgeon. My physiotherapist *Mári néni*, also visited him and she had often talked to me about him. For quite a long time I pretended to my class mates at school that he was my 'boyfriend' because I did not want to be left out of the conversations about boyfriends. He was a very handsome young man and good company. I could visit him in my wheelchair and we had long chats. Later we corresponded for some time. I enjoyed my time of freedom in the hospital. I was growing up and started to feel attractive and attracted to the opposite sex.

I was discharged from the hospital with my left leg still in plaster and because of that I did not return to the second year of Grammar school in the September of 1956 when I was 15 years old. The plaster which was to be removed six weeks after the operation was still there when the Hungarian Revolution broke out.

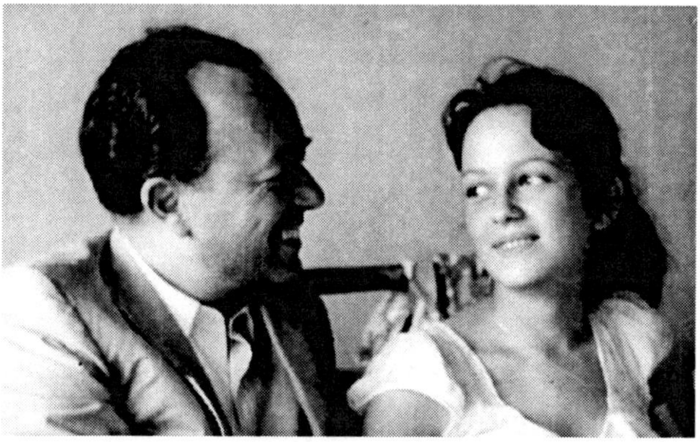

In hospital with my father after the operation in 1956

Chapter 9.

The Hungarian Revolution.

On the morning of Tuesday, 23rd October 1956, university students in Budapest posted flyers, with 16 demands, all over the city. They were demanding the withdrawal of Soviet troops, free elections by secret ballot, the removal of the hated statue of Stalin, the removal of all criminal leaders and a new government lead by *Nagy Imre*. The students declared their solidarity with the workers and students of Warsaw and Poland seeking national independence. When news of the Polish uprising reached Budapest the students decided to march to the statue of the Polish General, affectionately called "Father Bem" who fought with the Hungarians in the 1848 uprising against Austria. This was the first uprising in modern history against the tyranny of foreign rule, a revolution which united the landed gentry, peasants and intellectuals.

More and more people joined the demonstration carrying Hungarian National flags, Polish flags or plain red communist flags. When the workers left factories and offices in the afternoon they also joined the marchers. They cut the hated soviet emblem out of the centre of the red, white and green Hungarian flags. Soldiers ripped the five pointed soviet star off their caps. To the surprise of the demonstrators, the soldiers were joining them and were not going to fire on them! All over the city red communist stars were pulled down showing the people's wish to be free of Russian domination.

About 200,000 demonstrators gathered in front of the Parliament Building asking to hear the Prime Minister. They were not armed, and when the AVO officers asked them to disperse they shouted back "Down with the AVO! Pigs! Assassins!" They were asking for Nagy to appear and takeover the premiership. Nagy was a sixty year old, avuncular, Communist politician with no political ambitions. He loved good food and wine and made no secret of his view that Hungary need not follow the rule of Moscow. He was staying near Lake *Balaton* enjoying the annual wine harvest festival, and it took him some before he returned to Budapest. When he finally appeared on the first floor balcony and addressed the crowds, he promised reforms and asked the crowds to go home quietly. There was a silence and then Nagy asked the crowd to join him in singing the National Anthem.

At the same time another large group assembled in front of the Radio building asking for the student's demands to be broadcast on radio. The demonstrators decided to force their way into the building. First the AVO (State Security Department) men threw tear gas at the crowds and the soldiers in front of the building trained fire hoses on them. Then the first shots were fired. The AVO men opened fire on the crowd. Between one and two hundred men, women and children were killed, among them three Russian soldiers. Soon fighting broke out which was bloody and cruel. As a result a new Party leader *Kádár János* was elected. He promised the withdrawal of Soviet troops and asked the people to end the tragic fighting and senseless bloodshed.

We sat huddled round the radio trying to get some news. Hungarian Radio Stations only broadcast propaganda and to get reliable news we had to tune in to the BBC or Radio Free Europe which broadcast from Munich. These stations were heavily blocked by the communists to stop people listening to them. There were all kinds of noises trying to drown out the stations. In fact it was a punishable offence to tune into them and if the doorbell sounded while we had one of these forbidden radio stations on, not only did we have to turn off the radio but we also had to change the station.

In another part of the city, on a wide boulevard leading up to Heroes' Square, there stood an enormous bronze statue of Stalin, about 60 feet high. It was built after demolishing the beautiful church of Regnum Marianum, which was often visited by my mother before the war. Demonstrators tried to pull it down with ropes, but were not successful until metal cutting equipment was used to cut through the statue below the knees. The statue was pulled down and cut up. The head of Stalin was dragged through the streets of Budapest. Thinking about this reminds me of the similar destruction of the statue of Saddam Hussein which we watched while on holiday in Hungary in March 2003. It symbolised the end of tyranny and the beginning of freedom. We thought the battle was over but we were quite wrong.

The fighting continued the next day. Slogans appeared on shops and wall '*Ruszki haza!*' (Russians go home!) Normal life stopped, there was no school and no one went to work. There were Russian tanks everywhere. They were used to frighten the people, but tanks are not really suitable for street to street combat. They are vulnerable to attack by guerrilla fighters who threw 'Molotov cocktails,' petrol filled glass bottles with a cloth stopper which they lit before throwing them on the tanks.

In the morning jet fighters flew over the city and opened fire on demonstrators. Nagy was appointed Prime Minister as the crowds demanded but his first action was the announcement of martial law and the Government's request for soviet help to 're-establish order'. Later he denied that these were his decisions. It was evident that the Hungarian Army would not fire against the people; only the Russians and the secret police, the AVO, would. On the radio Nagy Imre called for calm and the laying down of arms in the interest of the future of the nation. Other broadcasters called the rebels 'pillars of fascism and a band of murderers, provocateurs, bandits and thieves'.

In the evening we covered our windows with blankets so that no light would be seen from outside and kept very quiet. I spent my time drawing and painting badges with the old Hungarian emblem to pin on our lapels. On the left hand side were 4 white and four red horizontal stripes representing the four rivers of old Hungary: *Duna, Tisza, Dráva, Száva* and on the right hand side the three hills of the Carpathian mountains: *Tátra, Mátra* and *Fátra* with the Apostolic double cross on the central hill showing that Hungary was a Christian country.

Food was scarce and my mother used what flour she had to make bread so that we had something to eat. My friend from school came to see us and my mother gave her some loaves to give to her brothers who were fighting at *Moszkva tér,* the large square which was about half a mile from our flat. We could hear the noise of fighting and we were very frightened. My friend asked if she could come with us to the west when we left Budapest, but my mother persuaded her to stay with her family.

Young men, some of them barely out of childhood threw Molotov cocktails at the tanks. Children spread oil soaked bales of silk on the road which immobilised the tanks and made them sitting targets for petrol bombs. Others managed to get rifles and were shooting at the Russian soldiers. Many were killed.

A group of people went to the British Legation to ask that the events in Hungary be discussed at the United Nations, but Sir Anthony Eden was busy dealing with the Suez crisis. The uprising spread across Hungary. At first the freedom fighters seemed to be winning and by the 30th October the tanks had retreated. People celebrated their victory over the Russians. The radio was taken over by people who promised to broadcast 'the whole truth and nothing but the truth'. There was euphoria everywhere. Complete strangers embraced each other in the street, crying with joy, hardly believing that Hungary would be free again.

The radio was broadcasting, asking for help from the West and Radio Free Europe from Munich encouraged the rebels to fight on until help arrived. We were falsely led to believe that the West would come to our aid. Hungary is a very small country compared with the USSR and had very little hope of winning.

Free elections were called for within 3 months. *Cardinal Mindszenty* was freed from prison after eight years and returned to his home in Buda. The fighting continued, many AVO men were rounded up and killed.

Two days later, on the 1st November, we heard news that the Russians were assembling a ring of tanks around the capital. Nagy called a cabinet meeting and Hungary's neutrality was declared. He cabled the United Nations but his cable was lost in the chaos over the Suez crisis.

Saturday, November the 3rd was a sunny winter day. People were returning to work, the general strike was over and the shops opened their doors for bread, potatoes and other essentials. The threat of famine was over. Negotiations started about the orderly withdrawal of Russian troops assisted by the Hungarian Army. The people believed that they had won a great victory. There were no Soviet soldiers to be seen in the city and there was a feeling of peace. Perfect strangers smiled and greeted each other with embraces, full of joy and hope for a better life. But their joy was short lived. On the 4th November at dawn, the tanks returned in greater numbers than before. The radio broadcast the news of the invasion. Later in the morning the Hungarian Writers appealed to the leaders of the world to help Hungary but by 8 o'clock the appeal became just SOS! SOS! SOS!

That evening *Nagy* was replaced by *Kádár*. The leaders of the uprising were rounded up and executed. The revolution was crushed and hope of freedom vanished. *Cardinal Mindszenty* took refuge in the United States mission. Thousands of people fled their homes to cross the Austrian border.

My mother realised that she now had an opportunity to leave Hungary. She remembered the last war, when the Russian soldiers entered houses and raped young women, like the fifteen year old Veronka and she was fearful that this might be repeated with her fifteen year old daughter Zsuzsi.

'If a Russian soldier tries to come into this flat, I will stand in the door and stop him. He will have to kill me first!'

She tried to convince my father that we should go to England. 'We have a 15 year old daughter. She could be raped by a soldier! What future does she have in this place? Going to university is out of the question for someone from our social class. Only children of workers and farmers get to university nowadays!'

She was very persuasive and very determined. She convinced my father and he agreed that we should try for a second time to escape from Hungary.

Chapter 10.

Second attempt to escape.

When my mother decided to leave Hungary, the whole family was against the idea. My father's brother and his wife tried to persuade us not to go. How could we leave all our possessions and go to a foreign land? How would we survive in a country where they spoke a different language? But my mother had lived in Paris for 3 years when she was in her twenties and she could speak not only French but English and German as well. Her brother Imre, now called Raoul had been living in London since 1930 and she had been longing to see him for the last 20 years. They had last met in 1936 when my parents and my grandmother Lotti spent two weeks in Paris on holiday, on a rather belated honeymoon, and he came from London to join them. She was sure that he would help us and welcome us.

My father was very close to his brother *Cincó* who tried to convince him to stay in Hungary. He asked him how could he leave his flat, furniture and everything that he had worked for? He could not even speak English, so what were his prospects of getting a job? He was 45 years old, a senior executive of a large company and he had his family heirlooms; paintings by his famous uncle, *Horváth József*, silver, furniture and paintings inherited from his mother, antique furniture, precious carpets and many books. Surely he could not leave it all behind? He was persuasive but my mother would not give up her plan.

Learning from the previous attempt, when my parents decided to leave separately and were glad that they had not lost everything when the attempt failed, my father decided that he would try to sell some of these precious possessions and turn them into small diamonds. These could easily be hidden on his person and brought later. But my mother, who was not attached to any of these possessions and wished that the bomb had exploded in 1945 in our flat, said that there was no time to lose, we had to go straight away. She was certain that if we delayed our journey, the border would be closed. So we piled several layers of clothes on ourselves and together left for the border town of Sopron near Austria, where we could stay with my father's uncle, the painter Horváth József and his wife. It was dangerous to travel, there were road blocks everywhere, so as my left leg was still in plaster, my parents managed to arrange for an ambulance to take us to the hospital in Sopron.

Several times during the journey we were stopped by armed guards, who peered into the ambulance to check that there were no fugitives in there. We showed them a letter that said that we had to go to hospital for treatment and seeing the plaster on my leg, they allowed us to pass. The journey took several hours and was very uncomfortable. In the hospital in Sopron, the plaster was cut open and then re bandaged, so that I could walk, but later I would be able to remove it myself. After being in the plaster for so long my leg was very stiff and painful.

The next day my father found a peasant farmer who came into town every week for the market, and asked him to help us across the border to Austria. He agreed to take us back to his farm on the next market day. A sum of money was agreed and a small picture was torn in half. My father had one half, and my mother would give him the other half as soon as we reached the border. He promised to get us across.

The following week we said good-bye to my father, and got on the farmer's cart. Our heads were tied with scarves to make us look like peasant women. We arrived at the farmer's mud hut in the evening where he was greeted by his hugely pregnant wife, surrounded by four or five little children. He sat down, took off his cap and took out a great big carving knife. He was completely bald and my mother wondered if our end had come! But he only used the knife to cut a piece of bread and cheese for his supper. We sat in silence and waited. Later two border guards arrived with their rifles and there was a hushed conversation in the entrance. We could not hear what they said and waited apprehensively. They came in and told us to follow them. As I was not very good at walking in my plaster, it was agreed that one of the border guards would carry me on his back while the other guard had both rifles. It was getting dark when we were taken outside and began the walk through the village. We had several layers of clothes to keep us warm and hardly any luggage. We did not carry a suitcase. When we reached a barrier on the road, the soldier put me down and pointed us in the direction of a small building.

'That way is Austria, just carry on walking!'

My mother thanked them and handed over her half of the small picture.

'Take this to my husband. He has the other half and when you give it to him he will pay you for helping us.'

So we set off into the dark night, along the bumpy road. I was holding on to my mother and leaning on my stick in the other hand. Every now and then there was a strong search light, which swept around. We were very frightened and crouched down low in the ditch, so as not to be seen. It turned out to be a tractor, which was ploughing the fields at night, or maybe looking for people to pick up?

Eventually we reached a small border station and my mother cautiously crept up the stairs and peered in through the window. I waited anxiously at the bottom wondering if we were in Hungary or Austria. She listened to the voices inside and realised that they were speaking German! So she plucked up courage and knocked on the door which opened and she asked in fairly good German for help. We were taken on the tractor to a school building, where several people were lying on the floor and settled down to sleep for the night when three men entered the room and one of them asked in Hungarian,

'Who would like to sleep in a hotel in Vienna tonight?'

Of course everyone wanted to go! They were all asking to be chosen. As we had just arrived and were on the floor nearest the door where they entered they saw my leg in plaster and said,

'We'll take this young girl and her mother'.

We went out into the night and got into the back seat of a small black car. My mother sat in the middle but the man next to her kept reaching over to me behind her back to try and touch me and she kept pushing him away. We were squashed in rather uncomfortably. I tried in vain to read the road signs and wondered whether we were really going to Vienna. Were they taking us back to Hungary? What will they do with us? We were very frightened and hardly dared to speak.

It was well after midnight when we arrived in Vienna. One of the men got out and made some phone calls. He came back with bad news, 'I am sorry but I can find no beds for you in a hotel.'

'Thank you for taking us this far, we will manage by ourselves,' my mother replied and we got out of the car, glad to be rid of the men who were acting suspiciously.

We started walking down the dark street. We didn't have to walk far until my mother found a hotel. We went in and she asked for a room for the night. I had never been to a hotel before and after our adventure it was wonderful to have a nice clean bed and a lovely room just for the two of us. It felt like heaven and we soon fell asleep.

The next morning my mother telephoned some friends who lived in Vienna. They came and generously paid for the room. We then found a room in a convent. The nuns looked after us and in the morning we were woken up by the smell of fresh bread and the sound of angelic chanting from the chapel. I stayed behind while my mother phoned my father and her brother to tell them that we had arrived safely and that she had some plans. She wanted to take me to Switzerland because she knew that rehabilitation services for polio were excellent there.

My uncle was very firm and told her to go straight to

the British Embassy and ask for asylum and she took his advice. While she was there she helped out with the registration of several refugees because she was proficient on the typewriter and the next day we got on a bus which took us from the Embassy to the railway station.

My mother said something to one of the officials as we were getting on the bus and he replied, 'Shut up!' I did not understand so my mother explained it to me. I was surprised to hear such language.

The journey took two days. At several stations the train stopped and we were greeted by people gathered on the platforms to give us chocolates, fruits and drinks which were very welcome and the train carried on its way in and out of tunnels through the Rhine region. I admired the view out of the window and tried to get some sleep at night on the uncomfortable bench.

Chapter 11.

Arriving in England.

After the long train journey we crossed the Channel by boat and arrived at Dover. We were permitted to land on the 2nd of December 1956 and were taken to the top of the hill to Connaught Barracks in Dover Castle with many other Hungarian refugees. People were sleeping in bunk beds in a large hall. They were all waiting to be interviewed. We were given some food which I had never seen before and I found very strange. Later I learned that it was baked beans and sausages. In the afternoon my mother managed to telephone her brother, my uncle Raoul, who arrived soon afterwards and whisked us away up to London in his Wolseley. He had to give the authorities his guarantee that he would look after us and that we were not communist spies. He had been helping with translating for refugees and was well known by the Immigration Staff that was why he knew that we had to register as soon as possible if we wanted to stay in England. We drove to London in his big black car and I was amazed to see so many strange sights!

I was fascinated by the little bright lights in the centre of the road. I had never seen anything like that before. My uncle told me that they are special to England and are called 'cat's eyes'. They were invented to help the cars to stay on the correct side of the road if the weather turned foggy and fog was common in England.

We stopped at a roadside restaurant for something to eat and drink and after travelling for about three hours arrived in London. The shop windows were all brightly lit up and stacked full of produce. In Budapest I was used to seeing almost empty shop windows and at night they were in darkness. Here neon lights shone everywhere, making everything bright and colourful. I did not know which way to look. I was turning my head left and right and getting quite dizzy, trying to absorb everything. The buildings looked very strange too; rows and rows of houses with tiny front gardens, standing right next to each other without any space between them and only two storeys tall. They looked almost identical but their style was unfamiliar to me.

In Budapest I was used to seeing large blocks of flats with four or five floors. In the country, houses were built on a single floor and were separated by gardens. They usually had iron railings in front and a ditch between the road and the pavement.

My uncle drove us to his house in north London. It was semidetached with bow windows in a long street with many other houses of the same design built in the 1930s. There was a small front garden and no garage. We were greeted by my aunt Joan and my two cousins Susan and Stephen. Susan was 2 years older than I was and we soon became very good friends. We had been corresponding with each other in the past and I felt that although an only child I now had someone I could look upon as a sister. Susan gave up her bedroom for us and moved into a little box room next door.

There were four bedrooms, Stephen, who was younger than I, had his own room next to that of my uncle and aunt who had the biggest one in the front of the house. It was quite difficult to communicate with my English cousins and aunt as I could not speak the language.

How I wished I had been a better student back in Budapest when my mother was trying to teach me. I often pretended to mislay my English book to avoid having a lesson. Eventually she gave up trying to teach me and found someone who came to the house to teach not only me but also my father. But I still had a very poor knowledge of the language. I had been learning English for only six months in Hungary.

I had never seen a television before. My uncle had a 12 inch set in a large brown cabinet which stood in the corner of the living room. I sat for hours watching it, concentrating hard and trying to understand what they were saying in the programs. I found the little bright light that glowed in the centre of the screen after it was switched off, quite fascinating and kept turning it on and off several times. This unfortunately ruined the set! I must be the last generation who grew up without television.

It must have been hard for my uncle's family to have two relatives from such a distant land suddenly arrive on their doorstep without any idea how long they were going to stay. Neither my cousins nor my aunt could speak any Hungarian. This made communication very difficult. When my aunt was going out and said 'I won't be long,' I thought she said 'I won't belong' which made very little sense. I also misheard the radio programme 'Sing Something Simple' as 'Sing Something Sinful' and wondered why it had such a strange title. English was a very puzzling language to me.

My uncle and aunt had a little brown 'sausage dog,' a dachshund called Maxi and I soon formed an attachment to him although I am not generally fond of dogs. My uncle teased him when he came home from work, by saying 'rhythm section' at which the dog started barking furiously. I have never found out what these words could have meant to him.

I had my first English Christmas in 1956 in London with my mother and my newly found English relatives. They had quite different customs from those I grew up with. There was the familiar tree but it was decorated many days before the 25th December and presents were not given until after the Christmas dinner. There was a large turkey, I had never eaten one before; nor had I tasted Christmas cake or Christmas pudding. I found it dark, bitter and horrible and I remember thinking, how could anyone enjoy it?

In Hungary I was used to a quiet festival celebrated on Christmas Eve. I never decorated the tree; I used to go out for a walk in the afternoon with my grandfather and the fully decorated Christmas tree appeared miraculously in the evening with the presents beneath. The tree was supposed to be brought by angels from the baby Jesus and their arrival was announced by little tinkling bells, usually after dinner, in the other room, which was out of bounds all afternoon. Then my father would say 'The angel has come with presents sent by the baby Jesus, let's go and see.' Then the door was opened and there in the darkness was the tree glowing with coloured lights. We sang Christmas songs and I was filled with wonder looking at the lights making coloured circles behind the 'angel hair'. After the presents were opened we went to bed and the next day was spent playing and reading and possibly going to church, although I cannot remember if we did or not. The only special Christmas food was carp fried in breadcrumbs on Christmas Eve. It had many tiny spiked bones which often stuck in my throat but I became an expert at removing them. It never stopped me from enjoying this special Christmas treat. It was usually accompanied by Russian salad (which in Hungary is called French salad), a mixture of diced vegetables with apples and cucumber in a thick sweet mayonnaise.

My mother tried to help my aunt with the cooking, but when she asked for 6 eggs to make a cake my aunt Joan was horrified. Eggs were very expensive in 1957 and a great luxury as it was not long after rationing had finished but we had no idea about the hardships people in England suffered after the war. To us it seemed that people had plenty of food. My mother was used to making different kinds of cakes from those in England. She had lessons from a famous pastry chef before the war and learnt to make light gateaux. Her favourite was a rich chocolate cake.

My mother started looking for work in London soon after Christmas. First she had to register as a Hungarian refugee and be given a work permit.

She had secretarial skills but her English was not quite good enough, so she signed up for evening classes to learn Pitman short hand and perfected her typing skills. She found a room in South Kensington and we would go 'shopping' in Harrods on Saturdays pretending that we could buy anything if we wanted to.

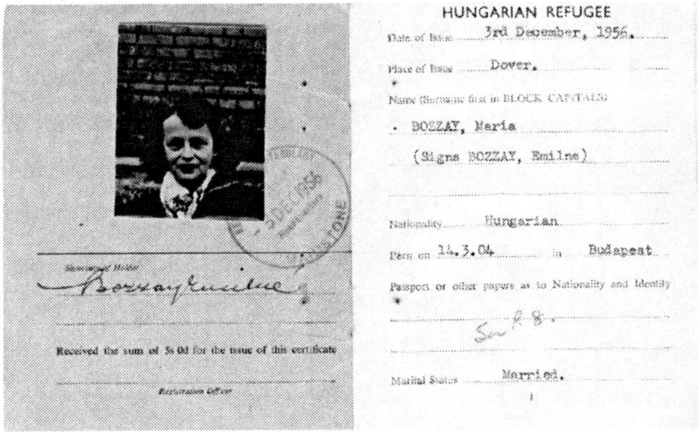
HUNGARIAN REFUGEE

Date of Issue 3rd December, 1956.

Place of Issue Dover.

Name (Surname first in BLOCK CAPITALS)

BOZZAY, Maria

(Signs BOZZAY, Emilne)

Nationality Hungarian

Born on 14.3.04 in Budapest

Passport or other papers as to Nationality and Identity

Marital Status Married.

Received the sum of 5s 0d for the issue of this certificate

Registration Officer

On the photograph in this permit my mother looks very confident and happy; her expression seems to show that she had finally achieved all that she had been planning for so many years. She had now become Maria (signing herself as *Bozzay Emilné* the 'né' meaning 'wife of') and interestingly gave her actual age of 52. She had to register with the police each change of address and was not allowed to accept any employment without permission of the Ministry of Labour.

Her first job was as a typist with the BBC in Bush House in January 1957 working for the Hungarian section. By the beginning of March she was working as a cook in the Clarence Coffee House in the City and a month later as Assistant Cook in Moorgate at the Kings Arm Yard where businessmen and office workers came for lunch. She learnt to make apple pies which she did every day, but she did not stay there long because on the 17th April she started to work for the Hungarian Weekly at Cumberland Court, Kensington. Her brother was not impressed that she kept changing her jobs but she knew what she was doing because while she was at the Hungarian Weekly someone came in looking for a typist and as a result on the 23rd May 1957 she found permanent employment with ICI (Imperial Chemical Industries) where she stayed until 1964. According to the 'Aliens Order of 1960' she did not have to be registered any more. She left her typist job at the 'Intelligence Department' of ICI just before her 60th birthday in case they forced her to retire and soon after found another job at the National Cash Register Company or NCR. Having changed her birth certificate by fifteen years she carried on working until 1979 when she officially retired at the age of 75 but only admitting to 60. Her boss, for whom she worked in the last months, was very pleased with her work and gave her a glowing reference.

Chapter 12.

School days.

In January 1957 my mother decided that it was time that I went back to school, but as I had been going to a grammar school in Budapest, she wanted me to go to a grammar school in England. My aunt Joan was very unsympathetic saying, 'Grammar school places in England have to be earned by passing the 11plus! My son did not get a place, so why should your daughter get one?'

My mother felt that we could not stay with my uncle and aunt much longer, so she took me to the Hungarian Chaplaincy in West London. This was a place where she hoped to get some help. As instructed we sat and waited until a tall nun came in and took her place behind a desk. She was dressed in a black habit with a strange hard semicircular bib on her chest, a white coif covering her cheeks and neck and a hard white plastic square over her forehead which was covered with a black veil. A rosary hung from her leather belt and there was a large silver cross on her chest. Her name was Mother Ursula. When she heard that we were looking for a school she telephoned the Reverend Mother Frances in Greenwich to ask her if I could go there. After a brief conversation she told us that I would be accepted as a boarder and it was arranged that I became a pupil in St Ursula's Convent School in Greenwich. But when we got up to leave the nun looked at me horrified and said to my mother, 'You didn't tell me that your daughter was disabled! There are many stairs in the school! I am not sure now that she can go there! I shall have to ring Reverend Mother again!'

My mother's heart sank in disappointment. It seemed that her hopes of finding a school for me were dashed. We waited anxiously for the end of the telephone conversation. Finally Mother Ursula said, 'Reverend Mother says that she will be even more welcome!'

And so early in February, I was settled in my little cubicle on the top floor of the school, in the dormitory which was divided from the Geography room by a very thin wall. The dormitory was large with 6 cubicles on each side of the room. One side had windows to the garden and on the other was the dividing wall. The partitions between the cubicles were only about 5 and a half feet high and there was a white curtain in the front which could be drawn to give a little privacy. We closed the curtains at night and in the morning Mother Joan who was French, came to wake us up would call, 'Are you visible?' and when we said yes, she opened the curtain.

Inside each cubicle there was a narrow iron bed with a few hard blankets which I found very difficult to arrange, especially if the bed had been stripped, as some of the nuns insisted should be done every morning. I was used to sleeping under soft light duvets but such luxuries had not yet arrived in England. There was a small corner cupboard set at an angle for a few clothes and a bedside cabinet on which I had the last picture taken of my parents and grandfather before we left Hungary. Above the cabinet there was a mirror and next to it a chair. The furniture was painted blue and cream.

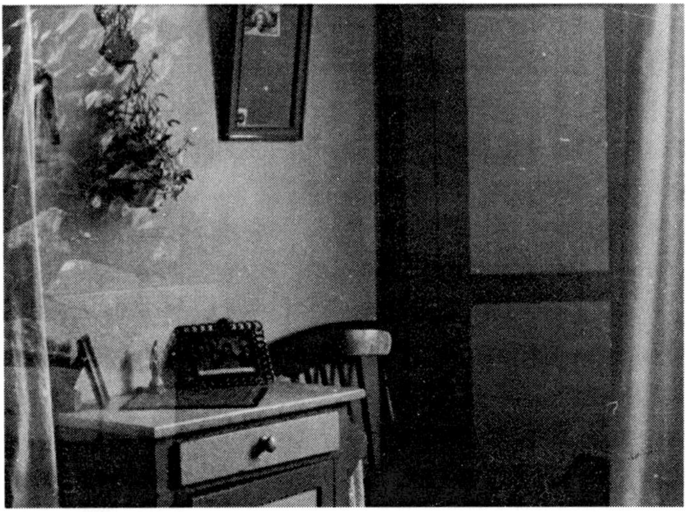

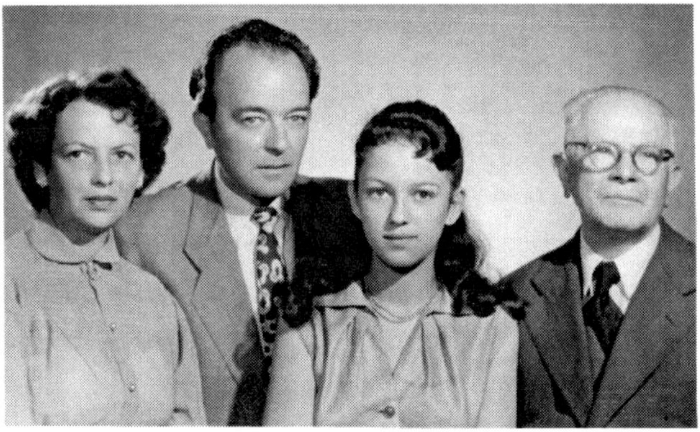

Last picture of my family in Hungary taken in May 1956

It was very cold in the dormitory, because there was only one radiator in this huge room and it was hidden behind a large chest of drawers. The windows were usually left open for 'fresh air' even in the middle of winter. This was to be my home for the next four and half years. It was a big change from a centrally heated, double glazed, comfortable flat in Buda. I missed my father desperately and getting him out of Hungary occupied my thoughts most of the time. I wrote to him two or three times a week and looked forward to his replies which helped me to feel close him and I prayed daily that he might come and join us soon. I made novenas, special prayers lasting nine days and tried to make sacrifices to hasten his coming, such as giving up sugar in tea, chocolates and even not having my hair cut until he came. I wanted to do everything possible to reunite our family.

In November 1958 my mother left her brother's house and found a room in 9 Neville Street, South Kensington where I was able to stay at weekends. Before this she used to come and visit me at the convent at weekends. She was always welcomed and often invited to stay for meals. The Reverend Mother put her in touch with the Labour politician Chuter Ede, who was Home Secretary until 1951 and whom she knew personally. My mother wrote to him as well as to the Conservative Prime Minister, Harold Macmillan, and several other MPs for help to get my father out of Hungary. My father wrote nearly every day and my mother and I replied almost as often. We numbered the letters in case one was stopped by the authorities or got lost.

I tried get up early every morning before breakfast to attend Mass in the beautiful little chapel and prayed hard that my father might be allowed to join us. Going to Mass was not compulsory but I felt that I wanted to do it. There is nothing like a tragedy to make one turn to God! Every day I joined the nuns who would kneel on both sides of the chapel in old oak choir stalls with hinged misericords, which were very hard and uncomfortable. They had brought them from France when they were expelled in 1907. They had even brought an altar which was eventually replaced in 1938 by the one I knew and loved. It was a delicately carved, lacy white marble altar in a gothic style. There were pews in the centre of the chapel for us, the congregation. At the very back of the chapel sat the Reverend Mother Frances Lemarchand and her 'deputy' the Mother Superior who also slept in one of the cubicles of the dormitory to look after us through the night.

Some of the nuns were teachers called Mothers and some were Sisters (with no teaching qualifications) who helped with the running of the convent. They worked in the laundry or in the kitchen, kept the place clean and were helped by a small group of Swiss au pairs and two girls from Thailand who had English lessons in return.

These Swiss and Thai girls came for one year and shared the dormitory with us. I became good friends with them. As I often heard my mother speaking German with our next door neighbour *Mrs Brüll* on the sixth floor of *Bajza utca* (who was like a grandmother to me and called *Brüllici*), the sound of German was not unfamiliar to my ears. As a result of this I picked up quite a lot of the Swiss German. Unfortunately there are several different dialects in Switzerland so I had to re-learn each time a new group of girls arrived.

I became a member of the class called Roper 3. There were three streams that year; Roper was the top stream, where we learned Latin. The less academic girls were placed in Martin where they learned useful skills like shorthand and typing and Ward was an extra stream because there were so many girls in that year. These names were derived from people who became martyrs and lived in medieval times when the Catholic Church was persecuted by Henry VIII.

To catch up with the Latin, I was given weekly private lessons by Reverend Mother Frances Lemarchand who had allowed me to come to St Ursula's as a boarder. She was very kind and gentle. These lessons took place in the parlour, which was a beautifully furnished room reserved for receiving visitors, with a large oak table in the centre, an antique sideboard and several comfortable chairs. I enjoyed my lessons and loved the Reverend Mother who was so kind to me. She called me Susie which was not really my name but she could not pronounce the Hungarian equivalent and I soon had to come to terms with most people calling me by this strange new name. In fact it was my mother who told them that my name was Susie when she first brought me to the convent. Maybe this was a conscious effort on her part to integrate me into English society.

I had an English lesson every morning in a little room at the top of the stairs next door to my classroom. My teacher was Mother Marie des Anges, a very talented German linguist. She could speak many languages even Hungarian, having spent 6 months in Hungary 10 years ago. She had been a missionary in her younger days in Alaska and Africa. I was lucky to have her all to myself and I made rapid progress. We talked only in English for about an hour each day. Mother Marie des Anges gave me 'homework' that took the rest of the day to finish. We raced though the *English Language for Foreigners* books by JB Priestley and soon I was beginning to understand what was going on in the classroom. In English lessons the class was reading Kidnapped of which I understood practically nothing at first.

The next book was Pride and Prejudice. Although I could not understand much of the story, I loved the sounds and enjoyed listening to the passages read by different members of the class.

As I had joined the class in the 3rd year I was a bit of an outsider. Friendship groups were already formed and I did not fit in. It is difficult to make friends without knowing the language and I was not a very outgoing person. Nevertheless I made friends with a girl called Sonia Shields, also a latecomer to the form. Sonia came from Grantham and she invited me to her house in Eltham one Easter holiday. The house was really cold but I appreciated the warm friendship she offered me. We kept in touch for some time after Sonia left school in the fifth form and married a GI from central USA. She met him while on holiday in Spain and she said it was love at first sight. She waited three years before marrying him and moving to the USA. I lost touch with her for many years and often wonder what had become of her and whether her marriage lasted since they hardly knew each other when they married. Recently we found each other again and she came to visit me. She has two grown up children and lives on her own, in retirement. The marriage was not a great success.

It was difficult to make friends, not only because I did not have the language but also because I was almost 2 years older than my classmates. I did not join them for lunch in the newly built dining hall which was at the bottom of the convent garden, down a long steep path. Instead I had my meals with the Swiss au pairs in a little dining room next to the kitchen in the basement of the main building. The people you eat with become your friends and I soon picked up the Swiss German dialect used by the girls. Unfortunately these girls only stayed for a year and each canton of Switzerland has a different dialect which I had to get used to. They were more my age and as we spent more time together we became closer friends. They also had English lessons with Mother Marie des Anges Dahmann, but not at the same time as I did.

Soon after I settled in at school, more Hungarian girls arrived at Greenwich until the little dormitory was full. First to arrive was *Margit Salát*. She was a very timid 12 year old girl who spoke no English. She came to England with her parents and her younger brother who was looked after by Barnardos. Her father had tuberculosis and he died soon after they came to England. Overnight Margit's hair turned grey. Later she became a Catholic under the instruction of the Hungarian nun, Mother Norberta who took her under her wing. Two sisters *Márta and Ildikó Kerékgyártó* arrived next; they were 13 and 11 years old and then *Maria Halász* who was 14 when she came to England with her brother *Jancsi* and their father. Finally there was *Ida* who thought that Adam and Eve lived in the 'tomato'. In Hungarian the word for 'Paradise' and 'tomato' are both *'paradicsom'*. She left Hungary on her own and soon returned because she was missing her family too much. The other girls had their families with them. All these Hungarian girls had English lessons together but I continued to have lessons on my own. I became very good friends with Márta and we played piano duets in school concerts. When I was in isolation with chicken pox we wrote to each other daily.

We had breakfast and tea in a separate little room near the library and two nuns were put in charge of us, Mother Ursula and Mother Joan. They took it in turns to sit with us while we were eating to see that we behaved nicely and they introduced us to the secrets of English etiquette and good table manners. These vary from country to country of course; for example which way to tilt the soup plate and where to place one's hands when not eating. We were told that these were important lessons to be learnt. Mother Ursula was typically English, tall and slim, who instead of walking, seemed to glide as if on skates. I thought she was strikingly beautiful. It was not the beauty of her face that struck me but her gentle manner and kind nature. It was as if the beauty of her soul shone through her face. It took my breath away if I met her unexpectedly round a corner in the corridor. She led the choir which I joined and I loved singing the hymns with the other choir members in the high balcony at the back of the chapel.

Mother Joan was the French teacher who was very jolly and lively. She had thick rimmed glasses. She was full of energy and always walked very quickly, almost running along the corridors. Born in France and passionately in love with the French language, she was a very popular teacher because she made lessons such fun. She helped me to catch up with extra lessons and I became quite fluent in French. Mother Joan could be found on the first floor in the French Conversation room next to Mother Anthony's, who was the Head Mistress. I would knock on the door and wait expectantly for permission to enter and I often helped her to make posters for displays. Mother Joan was in charge of missions and this often needed posters to encourage donations.

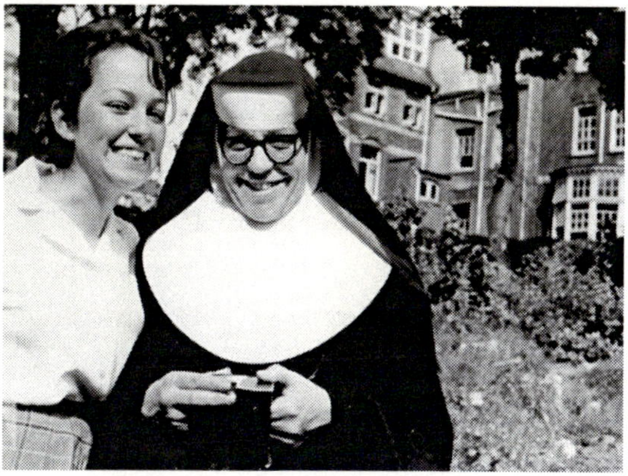
In the school garden with Mother Joan.

I put on weight rapidly due to the nutritious and plentiful meals we were given. We had a large cooked breakfast, a cooked lunch, tea with cakes and sandwiches and a cooked supper. The delicious food was prepared in a large kitchen in the basement under the direction of Sister Veronica with two or three other nuns and a Swiss girl. My mother always insisted that I cleared my plate. Food was relatively difficult to get in Hungary and we never wasted any. As well as sitting with us at meal times our Guardian nuns, Mother Ursula and Mother Joan also woke us up in the morning and settled us down at night. In this way they were a bit like a mother would be. I became very attached to them both especially to Mother

Joan. She and I were given violins and we started to teach ourselves at the weekends. We practiced in the art room because that was in the furthest corner of the school, so we were not overheard. Mother Joan had to wear a soft bib so that she could put the violin under her chin. As I already had piano lessons from another nun, Mother Cecilia, I spent much of my free time practicing in one or other of the rooms on a piano. There were several available in the school. Márta and Ildikó were already accomplished players and soon we were giving little performances in school concerts. Sometimes I played duets with Márta such as the *Berceuse* from the Dolly Suite by Fauré, which was used as the theme music for the radio program Listen with Mother. I was not very fond of this piece but my teacher insisted that it would be a good piece to perform at the school concert, so I persevered. I did not know anything about Listen with Mother. As we started to play the piece there was the gasp, just as it had been promised, from the audience. I also played the Bach Prelude 'Jesu Joy of Man's Desiring' which was used to accompany the *Ave Maria* which was also a very popular piece that I had never heard before. I loved having piano lessons but I was not entered for any exams because these were held in local centres and it would have been difficult for me to get there. My mother would have had to pay for the examination and she had little money to spare. My lessons were given to me freely, first by Mother Cecilia and later by the school's music teacher. I did not even have to pay for any sheet music I used. After the summer holidays I entered the 4th form (Year 10) and started to study for GCE O-level subjects in English Language,

Literature, Maths, Geography, Physics- with–Chemistry, French and Latin. I took the GCE Maths early, although I was struggling with the English units of measurement, I had already covered other areas in Hungary.

We also studied Religious Education but this was examined by a separate Catholic Examining Board. The Lower Certificate was GCE level and the Higher Certificate A-level. I passed both these with Distinction and received prizes for them. I was very much influenced by the kind nuns who looked after me. Their influence has affected me for the whole of my life and one of the most important events for me still, is going to Holy Communion. It sustains me and helps me to face any difficulties I might have. At the convent, I used to wait until all the nuns had been to Communion and then I was the last person, next to Mother Joan, whom I loved. This was an unspoken arrangement between us.

Mother Norberta, a Hungarian nun, arrived from France in 1959 and her methods were very different. I became very resentful when she looked though my drawer and left a note saying "I have seen it! Hm! Hm! M.N." I resented having my privacy breached and I started to compare her with the other nuns. They trusted me and encouraged me to strive to be better, not to live in insecurity and fear. I wanted to be trusted and would not disappoint them. Mother Eugenie was Irish and she often said 'Don't work too hard!' which made me do the exact opposite. I felt as the representative of my country and I wanted to prove myself and do my very best.

In the library I found a book about the Ursuline Method of Education. It was not meant to be read by pupils and I might have been in trouble if I was found looking at it. According to this book the mistress in the care of children should be 'supernatural', well balanced, kind, and firm, vigilant but discreet and prudent. Spiritual mothers should be like real mothers, loving their daughters with true, devoted charity, each one in particular. I copied out a passage from this book:

'Be kind and courteous to your daughters. When you reprove them, give them advice, urge them to do good and try to turn them from evil. You will obtain far more by kindness and affection than by harsh and severe words, which must be used only in case of necessity and then at the right time and place, taking account of the person with whom you are dealing. A spiritual mother has no domain in the conscience (only a priest does). She receives confidences and advises discreetly with frankness and supernatural spirit. The children feel this beneficent, purifying influence and the education is productive of true happiness'.

I felt that Mother Joan and Mother Ursula represented this ideal of an Ursuline Mother whereas Mother Norberta did not. St. Angela Merici who founded the order in Italy in the 16th Century wrote: 'Live and behave in such a way that you may serve as a mirror to your daughters, and begin by doing yourselves whatever you wish them to do.' I rebelled against Mother Norberta and would not do my homework with the other Hungarian girls. Mother Joan and Mother Norberta also fell out with each other as a result.

The awkward situation between us came to a head when the Reverend Mother, not the one who once taught me Latin, told my mother that I would have to leave! My mother was very worried and so was I but when I apologised for my rude behaviour, she forgave me and I was allowed to continue with my studies.

As I was so good at French, Mother Joan taught me to recite a piece from Horace by Pierre Corneille in which Camille a Roman girl pours out her resentment and hatred on Rome, having lost her lover in a fight with her brother. She hopes that the whole of Italy would be destroyed by all the nations and calls on a deluge of fire to rain down from heaven to destroy all its buildings and laurels and to see the last Roman take his last breath and then being the cause of all this destruction to die of pleasure!

I was entered for the national French Verse speaking competition. I successfully passed through the regional competitions and reached the finals which were held in South Kensington at the French Institute. The two of us, Mother Joan and I, travelled on the train and underground to South Kensington. This was quite a treat as Ursuline nuns live in an enclosed order and needed special permission to go out. Although Mother Joan was quite confident that I would win, another girl got the prize. According to Mother Joan the piece needed fiery expletives and determined courageous delivery. It was full of hatred against Rome and against Camille's brother, a Roman who has just killed her lover. Also the final 'e'-s, which are not pronounced in normal speech, had to be pronounced because it was verse. The girl who got the prize spoke in a whining voice as if crying false tears and did not pronounce the final 'e'-s. Mother Joan decided that the competition judges missed all these points and gave the prize to the wrong person. She arranged another competition to be held at our school as a consolation for me. I learned another poem from Andromaque by Racine and won first prize!

At the end of the school year there was a pilgrimage to Lourdes and I was asked if I would like to go. I have no idea how the cost of my journey was met, whether money was raised by the school or whether my mother contributed to the travel cost and the lodgings. We went by train and arrived at our hotel after the long journey. I was very impressed by the beautiful church and the grotto where many crutches and sticks were hanging, left by the people who were cured. I think there was a hope by some people in the school that I would be cured too, but I did not entertain such ideas. We had to go into a building where there were several small rooms with walk-in baths. I had to undress and put on a white cotton robe and enter the ice cold water. No obvious miracle occurred as I emerged from the water, but outside I saw several people on stretchers and in wheelchairs that were obviously so much more disabled than I was. It made me realise how lucky I was to be walking, admittedly with a stick but that did not matter to me. In the evenings there was a long procession and we joined the people with our candles in special holders, singing the Lourdes hymn with the refrain 'Ave, Ave, Ave Maria'. It was a very moving experience.

I did not like the shops that sold so much cheap religious merchandise, but I did buy a white marble statue of Our Lady holding the baby Jesus which I thought was very beautiful. My mother had given me the confirmation name of Bernadette, when I was 13, after Bernadette Soubirous who saw a vision in the Grotto of Lourdes of a Lady dressed in blue and white and was cured by the water which sprang up from the ground. My mother always hoped that we would visit Lourdes. Maybe she too was hoping for a miracle of healing, but no miracles happened. Instead I accepted my condition and did not expect to be cured.

I travelled to France again the following year at Easter, this time on an exchange to stay with the family of Isabelle Poirrier who had been to stay with us in England. Her father was an architect who worked from home and was able to take me out in his car every day to show me some of Paris. They lived in a large block of flats near the Arc de Triumphe. We saw the tomb of Napoleon, Montmartre, the Louvre, Notre Dame and all these were explained to me from an architectural point of view which was very educational and interesting. We did not go near the Eiffel tower because Monsieur Poirrier hated the sight of it and thought it was a blot on the landscape! After Easter they took me to their country house and on the way we visited the beautiful Chartres Cathedral.

It took my breath away to see the enormous Cathedral and the large round stained glass window with its jewel-like colours of intense red and blue. I thought it was the most beautiful cathedral that I had ever seen. We also went to Versailles where I had my picture taken sitting on a chair at the top of the stairs overlooking the beautiful gardens. I had a wonderful time in France and my French was much improved, mainly because of the help of Isabelle's 7 year old little brother Jean-Jacques.

Isabelle also had an older sister who was studying at the Sorbonne and she took me with her on a memorable day to attend one of her lectures. I sat in the stepped wooden seats of the lecture theatre but I cannot remember what the lecture was about.

I also visited one of my mother's Hungarian friends, who lived with her husband, a consultant doctor, in a beautiful flat in Rue St Honoré, a very select road. I was invited to dinner and she had a butler, which I thought was very strange. He came round offering me the various dishes and would not move the dish away until I took as much as he thought I should have. I was given presents for me and my mother. The three weeks of Easter holidays soon came to an end and shortly afterwards I had to sit my GCE exams. I passed all the subjects but I did not do particularly well in English language. I scraped through the Latin but my best mark was in French! I had passed Maths the year before.

Although I did not study French at A level I kept up my French studies and attended some of the classes when possible. I decided that I would study Chemistry and not French at University because that would lead to a job. So I chose to study Pure Mathematics, taught by Miss Murphy, who was Irish, and Applied mathematics with Miss Loftus. They were both very good teachers although Miss Murphy did have a habit of banging on the top of my head with her knuckle if I made a mistake, saying 'You silly goose!' Miss Loftus was very gentle and kind. She had no children of her own but looked after her two nieces who had lost their parents. One of them, Margaret Howard was in my class, her sister was two years older. I also wanted to study Chemistry and Physics. Unfortunately our Chemistry teacher became ill in the second year of our A-level studies and no replacement could be found so we were given a syllabus and told to get on with it on our own, which we did! The Physics teacher was useless. She was in her late 70's and had retired long ago. She had a bad memory and usually forgot the 'proofs' of equations saying, 'I could do it last night!' There were 8 girls in the class who were studying Physics and I was the only one who passed, thanks to the private tutor my mother found for me, who came to the house at weekends.

I passed all my A levels, as well as the Higher Religious Certificate with Distinction and I applied to the Imperial College in South Kensington to study Chemistry. I was asked to attend an entrance exam and an interview. The entrance exam was mainly an intelligence test which I was not good at, as English is not my mother tongue and it consisted largely of word puzzles. I was interviewed by three men who asked me if I had any intentions of getting married, and even if I had a boyfriend! Out of the 150 applicants only 30 students were taken and not one of them was a girl! I was devastated and planned to retake my A-levels at the Croydon Technical College so that I could try my luck the following year. But the admission officer told me that I would be wasting that year and as I had perfectly good A-level results I should try to study either at East London or the Northern Polytechnic.

I travelled to London on the train and found the first College in a very run down part of East London. I was interviewed and told that they were very happy to take me and would even start a Chemistry course for me if I decided to come! I was not impressed with this college and I cried bitter tears on the bus back to Charring Cross.

At the Northern Polytechnic I was interviewed by the principal, Dr. Gerrard who asked for my details and I was enrolled straight away to start in the September of 1961. It was as easy as that with no entrance exams and no awkward questions about boyfriends. This College offered internal London University Degrees, which meant that the students were not examined by their own lecturers but by lecturers of London University, which then granted the degrees. At the end of each year we had to go to Central London to be examined in Chelsea Town Hall, together with a large number of other students from other Colleges. It was in fact more difficult to pass these exams because our tutors had no inside knowledge of the questions.

Chapter 13.

Starting College.

My uncle Raoul offered me accommodation while I was studying at the College. It was a few stops on the underground from Holloway Road to Bounds Green, then one stop on a bus or a long walk to his house. This time I was given the little room and Susan, my cousin, stayed in her own room. She introduced me to cigarettes which were not really allowed by her parents or mine. In fact her brother Stephen was offered a large sum of money, £21, if he did not smoke until the ripe old age of 21! I am not sure if Susan's parents knew of his or her smoking. As they both smoked heavily they probably could not detect the smell on anyone else. Sadly Raoul died of smoking related cancer in 1972. His wife Joan who also smoked heavily lived into her eighties although her health was very bad due to smoking.

I started College in September 1961. I sat three rows up from the front of the stepped lecture hall next to the only other girl, Kathy Hull, in the class of about thirty. When the register was called I heard the strange name, Michael Snarey, and turned round to see the owner of this name. It belonged to a ginger headed boy with pale eyebrows and lashes and intelligent blue eyes. He also had a very nice resonant voice. Later in the day when we were standing in the Physics laboratory and were asked to choose a partner for practical work in Physics, Kathy and I decided not to choose each other but pick one of the boys. I boldly went up to Michael and asked him if he was good at Physics practicals because I felt that he was not the kind of good looking boy my mother warned me against but someone I could trust and he modestly replied that he was not too bad. This was my lucky day and we soon became very good friends.

Kathy chose a boy called Dick Lee, because she thought he was good looking but it turned out later, that he already had a girlfriend and was not interested in her romantically. Kathy, Michael and I became the best of friends and another boy called Malcolm joined us to make a foursome. Michael and Malcolm were Sandwich Course students who spent six months in college and six months working. We spent our lunchtimes in the buffet of the college, I usually had a roll and a Penguin or a Kit-Kat, but when it was one of our birthdays we celebrated at the local Chinese Restaurant. At this time Michael had a girlfriend called Heather, a tall attractive girl he was working with at the Tropical Products Institute. She was very keen to get engaged, but they kept having arguments. It seems that Michael had already decided to end that relationship when he met me.

I enjoyed the lectures and found the subjects very interesting. Organic chemistry was taught by an elderly lecturer called Dr. Finar whose head was bent sideways because of a stiff neck. He wrote an excellent organic chemistry text book that we used and because he had three daughters, he frequently made derogatory remarks about women, he was a real misogynist! I do not think he would get away with such remarks nowadays, but he thought it very humorous. The Inorganic chemistry lecturer was a lean, dark, good looking man, John Bull. He spoke very quickly and it was difficult to take accurate notes of everything he said as he walked up and down in front of the blackboard. I was very keen to do well in this subject because I wanted to impress him, so I made a special effort to learn all the given details. I especially liked it when he was talking about the parts of the atom and he described the mass of the electron as a fraction of the mass of proton as being one thousand eight hundred and fortieth- *approximately*!

Dr Norbert Singer was our lecturer in thermodynamics. This was a difficult subject needing all our concentration which was sometimes lacking. Once when Kathy and I were giggling about one of the boys sitting in front of us and not paying attention to the lecturer, he turned and said 'You make me feel as though I had lost my trousers!' He thought we were laughing about him! However he was a very good lecturer and eventually we understood the subject.

There were long chemistry practicals in an old laboratory. These took all day, but we were able to go for tea and lunch breaks in the canteen. It was more like following a recipe making new compounds or identifying some unknown compound. To purify the crystals that we had synthesised, we had to wash them in a suction filter pump which was attached to a tap of fast flowing water. As the water flowed through a small valve the air was sucked from the side arm of the filter flask which speeded up the filtering process. We were told never to mix solvents with concentrated nitric acid in the filter flask, but one day I mixed a solvent with concentrated sulphuric acid. Nothing at all happened for several hours but when I returned from my lunch break I noticed that the mixture had started to bubble and boil furiously. I watched fascinated wondering what caused the reaction to start so suddenly when the whole filter funnel exploded showering all those nearby with concentrated sulphuric acid! One of these was poor Michael, who worked on the opposite bench. We all dashed to the sink and drenched ourselves with water to wash away the acid and luckily no great harm was done, but I realised how inadequate I was at practicals and how much better Michael was. He had been working in a chemical laboratory for some years and had plenty of experience, whereas I did not even have a proper chemistry teacher at school for the last six months and had no practical experience.

During the long summer holidays I found a job in the laboratory of the British Coal Utilisation Research Association in Leatherhead. My parents worried about me working and how I would travel there on the train but I did not have any doubts about managing. I still walked slowly with a stick and had a slight limp but that did not stop me from doing what I wanted to. Every morning I caught a train from South Croydon Station and worked under the direction of a young man called Brian. He had a diffident air and to instruct me he used to say, 'If I were you I would do it this way,' or 'I wouldn't do that if I were you!' I carried out several important experiments with coal samples. I was introduced to the art of glass blowing and had to work on different samples of coal dust to find their surface area. This involved placing a weighed sample of coal dust in a glass bubble, which I had to make by glass blowing and attach it to the vacuum line. After all the air was evacuated I removed the glass bulb by sealing the tube leading to it with a blow torch, broke it in a solvent contained in a special thermos flask and measured the rise in temperature. From this measurement and knowing the mass of the coal dust, I had to work out its surface area using a calculator with a crank handle. Electronic calculators were yet to be invented.

As my father had sent me a very good 35 mm single lens reflex camera I became interested in processing and developing my own pictures. There was a dark room down the corridor from where I worked and I found someone who was willing to teach me how to use the dark room. After I was married we bought our own enlarging equipment and were able to develop pictures at home.

At this time I earned just over £9 a week which had to be collected on Fridays from the cashier in a small brown envelope. It seemed a fortune to me. I bought my first beige leather handbag for £3 and felt very grown up using it. I worked in the laboratories in the following two summer holidays. Travelling on the train I met a nice young man and after several days he started talking to me. When he found out that it was nearly my birthday he invited me out to dinner! This was my first date and I was very excited. We went to a restaurant in Streatham, and later he took me to my first Chinese Restaurant. He lived on a houseboat on the Thames and I have no idea where he worked or what he did but he seemed very nice. I seem to remember that he took me out only three times and then finished the relationship, which was a little disappointing. This was my first rejection and slightly dented my ego.

In the college library where I studied for many hours I spotted a good looking young boy sitting opposite me wearing mustard coloured corduroy trousers. I kept looking at him and wishing that he would ask me out and eventually after a few days he did. He was a dental student, called Chris Littler and he had a little black old fashioned Ford car. He lived at Ilford, a good half an hour's drive from the college and he very kindly gave me a lift to Brownlow Road, where I lived with my uncle and aunt, even though it was not on his way home. After several weeks of this daily detour he invited me to his home for tea and introduced me to his parents. I felt that the relationship by now was getting serious. His mother opened the front door and as I tried to enter, I slipped and fell flat on my face into the hall! They had a wide shiny copper door step. I was very embarrassed, and felt that I had not made a good impression! After tea Chris took me up to his bedroom where he played and sang on his guitar a song about a gypsy. The relationship did not last. It was hardly a relationship at all and soon afterwards he resumed the friendship with his former girlfriend. I did not get a ride in his new car, a Hillman Imp which he had won in the University raffle, by guessing how far it would travel on a gallon of petrol.

I had another boyfriend from Libya, a mathematics student, called Ashim. He was very good looking but I soon realised that he was a Muslim and when he returned home, he could possibly decide to have more than one wife! Not as if we ever discussed marriage but I did not like the idea of being married to a Muslim, so broke off the friendship.

I was also taken out a few times by one of my class mates Julian who borrowed his father's car and took me to Hampstead Heath to a restaurant. He liked mountain climbing and was quite athletic but I was not too keen on him either.

At the end of the first year of college I asked my mother if I could invite some friends for a party and she agreed. About ten people came, Kathy and of course Michael with his girlfriend Heather. Michael brought his record player which he left behind at the end of the party, either accidentally or on purpose so that he could come back for it the next day and ask me to come with him to Brighton. He took me on his motorbike with a sidecar and we had a lovely time. We were walking along the seafront and Michael asked me if I would like to have children, and if so, how many? I replied that I would like six or eight or as many as happened to come along! This was the result of my convent upbringing and not a seriously considered decision. Luckily my answer did not seem to have put him off altogether, because we continued to see each other all through the summer and at the end of the summer holidays we got engaged on my birthday. We chose a ring with a red ruby in it and my mother insisted that Michael went down on his bended knee in front of me to ask me to marry him in her presence and that of his parents! Only a month or so before I told Michael that we were just good friends and on no account would I marry him! When we returned to college no one guessed to whom I was engaged! I kept it a well guarded secret although Kathy and some other close friends knew.

In the November we had the unbelievable but very happy news that after six long years my father was finally coming to England. He had applied for permission to leave Hungary every six months, thirteen times in total. When he was refused, he had to wait six months before he was allowed to apply again until finally he was granted an exit paper, not a passport, and an entry visa to England. We were very excited, and thankful to whoever it was that interceded on his behalf. Since my mother wrote so many letters to so many different people, it was impossible to know which one was responsible for this miracle. It did seem like a miracle! In six years I had grown up and became an independent young woman. I was only a fifteen year old child when I last saw him.

My father was called in to the Ministry, told that he was a lucky man and he could leave Hungary to join his family in England. He was allowed to take not only his personal possessions but even an allowance for my mother and me who had left illegally. Everything had to be itemised in great detail and valued, as the limit was quite low the items had been given little value by the kind assessor. Then it was put in large containers called 'lifts' and loaded onto a train to be brought to England.

We travelled to Dover with my uncle Raoul to meet him and it was a very joyful reunion. I cried tears of happiness when I embraced my Daddy and my parents hugged each other. During the six years separation my parents had to lead independent lives and they needed a lot of readjustment to get used to living together again. My mother was working in London at the Intelligence Section of ICI and my father eventually found a job at the quality control laboratories of Philips in Croydon. He bought himself a little beige Minivan.

At College, Michael and I sometimes missed practical sessions and instead went to the cinema or to the Ideal Home Exhibition and as a result I failed my organic practical exam at the end of the second year. This was partly due to the fact that the exam was in an unfamiliar laboratory in Chelsea and all the necessary chemicals had to be requested from the far end and partly because I was so bad at practicals. I soon became very tired from walking up and down the large room and I was also slow. I was given the chance of a retake the following year, when I asked if my bench could be nearer to the store cupboard and so I passed the exam at the end of the third and final year. However this time I failed my physics practical! It was on the day when Michael and I were due to go on holiday on the Norfolk Broads in a boat called Dazzling Waters with Michael's two sisters, Babs and Tina, Babs's husband Richard and two of their friends. I could not concentrate on the practical exam. I was so excited! I went straight to the train station from the exam to travel up to the Norfolk Broads. We had a wonderful week. I shared a double bed on the boat with Tina and Michael slept in the prow, but very early in the morning we would wake up and creep out while everyone was still asleep to go for a row in the dinghy that was attached to our craft. We would go fishing and come back for breakfast hours later when the rest of the party was just waking up having missed the best part of the day!

As Michael was doing a sandwich course, the 3 year course took him 4 years. He attended college for six months and worked for six months. I also had to retake my Physics Practical and I was not awarded my degree until a year later. This was why we waited until the August of 1965 when exam results were announced before we got married, although the wedding was planned for that date because we were certain of passing.

In 1964 after I finished university I got a job at the laboratories of the Gas Council at the end of the Fulham Road travelling there every day from my home in Croydon. It was a difficult journey so my boss kindly found someone who came by car from the same area and my father took me to a meeting point. It still took about an hour each way. To avoid the heavy traffic, my kind driver used to leave at about four o'clock and I had to go with him! I enjoyed my work, putting the nasty smelling mercaptans into natural gas and finding out the smallest amount which could still be detected. Natural gas has no odour so users might not be aware of a gas leak quickly enough which could result in an explosion. Mercury was used in manometers to measure gas pressure and I spent quite a lot my time clearing up spilt mercury droplets from the floor as most of the other workers did not think it was worth bothering about. Not only is it detrimental to health, it also forms an amalgam with the gold in wedding rings. The image that many people have of the mad scientist was often the result of mercury poisoning.

I made friends with a young girl, Pat who worked in

the basement in a very small room where the hazards of mercury vapour were much more relevant. Pat was about my height, quite short and nearly ten years younger but she was already married and was very knowledgeable about all sorts of things including birth control. She accompanied me to the Family Planning Clinic to get advice before I was to get married. I would not have dared to cross the threshold there on my own, but I knew that I would not be in a position to have children while Michael was studying for his MSc in Norwich and I was the sole breadwinner.

Pat told me that had a wonderful husband called Jim, who was a chemist and very clever and able in every way. From her description I imagined him as a tall broad shouldered muscular man who could do anything. So I was very surprised when having been invited to dinner in their Streatham flat he turned out to be just a little taller than Pat. I cannot remember what we had for dinner but I am sure it was delicious as Pat was a very good cook.

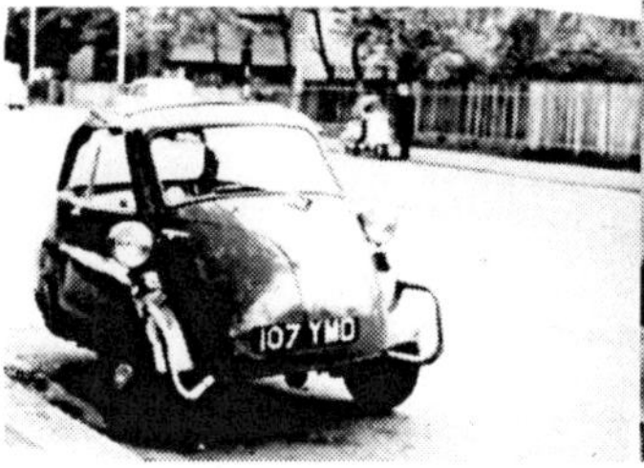

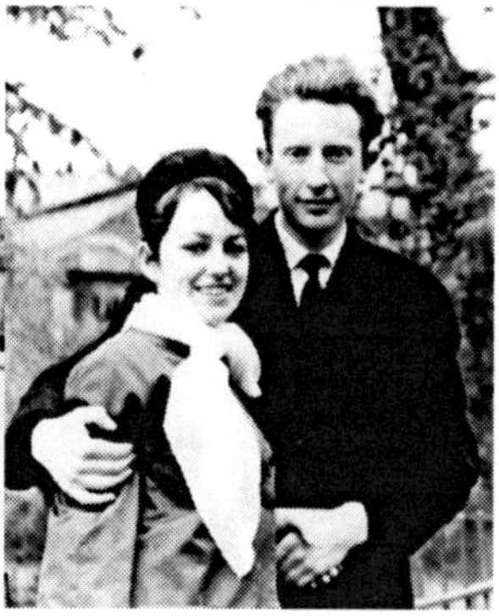

Chapter 14.
Getting married.

In the evenings after coming home from the laboratory of the Gas Council, I started to make my wedding dress. I bought the material in Oxford Street at £1 a yard. It was artificial silk and I needed ten yards for the Vogue Couturier pattern, which featured on its cover the beautiful model Jean Shrimpton. The dress was designed by John Cavanagh, a London designer and was worn by the Guinness girl who got married that year. It had a slim princess line, three quarter sleeves, a stand up collar and a very long train attached from the shoulder. First I tried out the pattern in a floral cotton fabric and made a short summer dress just to see if any alterations were needed. I bought long white elbow length leather gloves and ordered a pair of white boots from Anello and Davide, just off Oxford Street, which were a copy of the latest French fashion by Courrège having cut-out tops and a little bow in the front. None of this was visible under the long wedding dress but I could wear them for many years afterwards and feel fashionable. I also spent some time making some embroidered sheets for my "trousseau". They were to fit a five foot bed which I imagined that we would have, but we ended up in sleeping on a three foot single bed in our first flat!

The night before the wedding Michael and I made the sandwiches while my mother prepared sausage rolls and other finger food. I had already bought the cake from a famous Fulham baker shop which I saw advertised in the Weddings magazine, for the extravagant price of £18! This was the most expensive item of the whole wedding. It had three tiers with pink sugar roses for decoration and real live fern. After the wedding I stored the two upper tiers in a cardboard box in the airing cupboard where they soon developed a layer of mould and had to be thrown away. In the same way my lovely wedding dress which my mother put in the flower box became mouldy.

There were no hen parties or stag parties and no hairdressers or 'makeovers.' I got dressed and waited for the car to take me and my father to the church for 3.30. I could not understand why the driver took such a roundabout route, but he explained that the bride had to arrive a little late! It was a lovely wedding, a friend who was a professional photographer and his wife whom I had met at the Croydon Camera Club took the photographs and afterwards the small party assembled in our garden. Our guests were some of Michael's large family and all my family in England, as well as our friends. Michael's sister Tina was my bridesmaid, as she already had a suitable dress, and Michael's best friend Alex was the best man. There were photographs in the garden and cutting of the cake in the flat. I do not think there were any speeches, but I have a picture of Alex reading a few telegrams.

Afterwards we left to go to our new first floor flat in Fulham. I found it from a local advert. It was within walking distance from my work and this was its only virtue. Michael and I spent two or three days cleaning it and lifting up and throwing away layers and layers of lino with several old hairpins between the layers. There were two single beds in the living room which we tried to push together but they kept moving apart and in the end we decided that it was more comfortable to sleep on just one than to keep falling down between the two. So much for the plans for my five foot bed! We have often repeated sleeping together on a single bed during our married life and found it quite comfortable.

The toilet was outside and to reach it we had to go down a long flight of stairs. The second room was the kitchen as well as the bathroom. It contained a table and two chairs and a stove on a pedestal which made it just a bit too tall for me and a bath covered with a piece of hardboard. I was quite ashamed of our accommodation and would not allow my parents to see it or invite any friends there, but it suited us because we could afford the rent.

The following Wednesday we left for the Scilly Isles for a week's honeymoon. We travelled by train to St Ives and from there by helicopter to St. Mary's. We had a lovely honeymoon in a small hotel in St Mary's, the capital. We drank mead, the drink made with honey for honeymooners. One morning Michael went out to buy his usual Guardian newspaper and met the Prime Minister Harold Wilson out for a walk and they said good morning to each other. Mr. Wilson always went to the Scilly Isles for his holidays.

We took a boat trip to the uninhabited twin peaked island of Samson. The boat ran ashore and we had to jump into the water to get to the deserted beach. There was not a single person to see. The water was a bit chilly even for August, too cold to swim in. We had the whole day to explore the island which was wonderful. The boat did not come back until the afternoon. We returned with a large granite pebble as a souvenir.

Another day we visited Tresco which has a wonderful tropical garden with huge exotic plants, succulents and beautiful flowers. On one of the other islands, St. Martin's, we stopped where we saw a sign on a gatepost advertising teas. The elderly lady serving tea looked at me very strangely and then asked Michael what happened to 'his sister's' leg. She was surprised to learn that I was his wife and not his sister!

After our short week we had to return to St Ives by boat because the helicopter could not take off from the island due to bad weather conditions and soon we were back home in the little rented flat.

We were not there for very long however because at the beginning of October Michael started to work for his MSc at the University of East Anglia under Professor Alan Katritzky and I found a job at Mackintosh's chocolate factory. I did consider teaching science as a last resort, and wrote a letter of application but did not even receive a reply from the Education Department in Norwich. Maybe there were no vacancies. I also had an offer of a job as a personal assistant of Professor Katritzky but Mackintosh's paid better and I was the whole of the 'research department'.

Not long after I started work I was joined by a glamorous new research assistant, Avril Griffiths. She looked like a film star with her long blond hair in a fashionable high bun and we soon became very good friends. She came from Blaenevon and was shortly to be married in Wales to Monte. To our great surprise we found out that both she and Michael were born in the same Nursing home, Llanfrechfa Grange near Cwmbran, although not in the same year, but some seven years apart.

We spent many months working together and when there was not much work we planned menus, dinners and sweet dishes for our husbands. I worked at the labs for three years while Michael studied for his MSc and then his PhD. We drove round in a yellow three wheeler Reliant Robin which was great fun although very noisy. It was a great improvement on the little red bubble car we had previously. There was a small slope to the parking place outside our one bed roomed flat with a brick wall facing the parked cars. Michael used to play the game of speeding down the slope and then stopping suddenly. One day his foot slipped and the front of the car hit the brick wall! The large hole in the fibreglass body cost £18 to repair, quite a large sum of money in those days when my monthly salary was less than double that amount. The same as the cost of the wedding cake two years before!

One day as I was returning from work I saw a man knocking at our front door. I asked him what his business was and he said that he was acting as a car salesman but really he was a driving instructor. I wondered if he would be able to teach me to drive even though I had a paralysed left foot, and he offered to try and help if I came into the showroom. The car on which I learned to drive was a Fiat 850 and the clutch was adapted in such a way that I could depress the pedal using my whole leg. I had twenty driving lessons after which I failed the driving test. I felt completely despondent but my instructor encouraged me and promised that he would arrange for me to take the test again four weeks later. This was amazing because in those days it was difficult to get a date for a driving test so quickly. Sometimes people had to wait months before retaking it. He also told me that as I was twenty four years old I would need four extra lessons. But he was right, four weeks and four more lessons later I passed. Even before my husband who was still driving using a motorcycle licence! But he did not need many lessons in order to pass first time.

We were ready to buy our first car. With Michael's grant which was paid at the beginning of each academic year, we purchased a dark blue Singer Chamois, the luxury version of the Hillman Imp for £595. It had some walnut trim inside and even a radio. We were very happy!

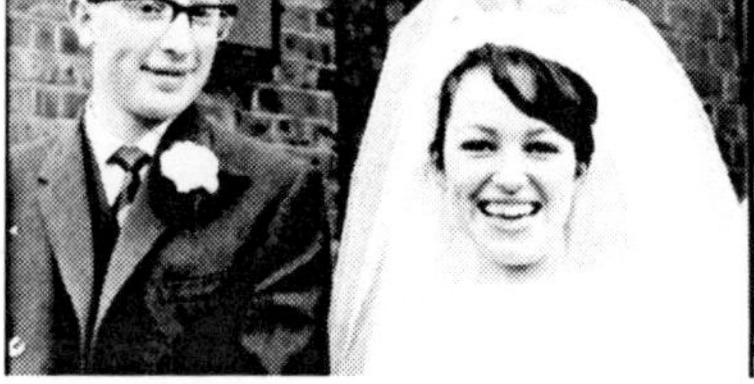

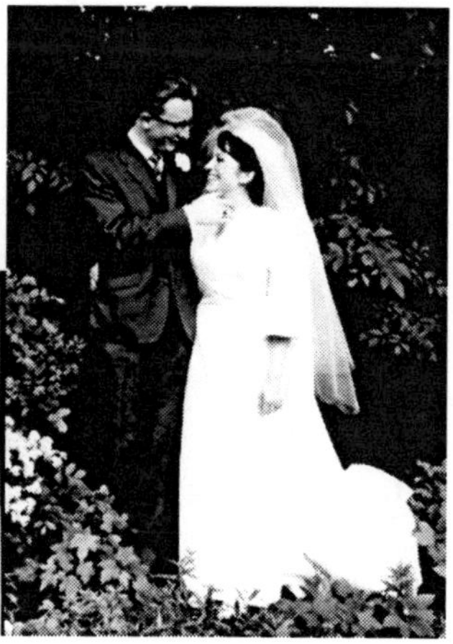

Chapter 15.

Return to Hungary.

In 1967 we started to make plans to visit Hungary. First we needed a passport and I also had to become a British subject. As my husband was British this was no problem. After I had placed a notice in the local paper for three consecutive weeks in case anyone had any objections, all I had to do was to find a Notary Public in front of whom I could swear allegiance to the Queen.

Having the necessary papers, we applied for our joint passport. I was too frightened to travel to Hungary with separate passports in case they decided to retain me and put me in prison for leaving the country illegally. We booked a package holiday for the end of August, staying one week by the Balaton in the popular town of *Siófok* and one week in Budapest at the Palace Hotel, the cheaper option. The plane from Heathrow was an old Russian Ilyushin turboprop with very little leg room but the food during the flight was very good. We were offered fresh bread, Hungarian salami and cheese followed by grapes.

We arrived after dark in Budapest, as the long flight had been delayed. At the passport check my heart was beating very fast and my knees were trembling as Michael handed over our joint passport to the official who looked very swarthy and looked at me inquisitively. I refused to answer him in Hungarian. After what seemed like an age he handed the passport back and we were allowed to pass. Further on people were called to come this way in Hungarian and again I refused to show that I understood and did not move. All those who came forward had their bags thoroughly searched, including their handbags and purses. It was not allowed to take in any foreign currency. When the same call came in English we moved forward and our bags were not searched, just marked with a chalked on cross. We were illegally smuggling in a short wave radio which we hoped to convert to useful Hungarian currency on the black market. Radios like this were much sought after as they could receive programmes from the West such as Radio Free Europe and the broadcasts by the BBC. Radios sold in Hungary were made so that these wavelengths were not available. The tourist rate of exchange even then was much more favourable than the "official" rate of exchange, but it was more profitable to take a radio for sale.

We were transferred to our hotel by an ancient *Ikarus* bus which was a real boneshaker! The bus driver disengaged the gears and freewheeled down any available slope in order to save fuel. This is not only illegal in England but also very dangerous.

The hotel was a short distance from the lake and the accommodation was fairly basic but comfortable. In the morning we were served what is known in Hungary as an English breakfast, ham and eggs while we saw the Hungarians drinking *pálinka* and eating cold meats, salami and cheese. One member of our party, an Indian lady who was Jewish by religion, tried to explain that she did not eat pork. As I refused to admit that I could speak or understand Hungarian, Michael tried to help saying in his broken Hungarian, '*Nem disznó hús*'. (No pig meat).

Eventually I could bear it no longer and spoke to the waiter explaining the problem. He was amazed and overjoyed, 'Why didn't you say that you were Hungarian! My wife works in the kitchen! What is your favourite food?' And from then on we had special treatment such as salami and Hungarian sausages for breakfast; we were even offered the customary *pálinka*, a very strong plum brandy, which we refused.

The next day another waiter leant over and whispered in Michael's ear 'Vilkinson?' Michael replied, 'My name is Snarey, I don't know Mr Wilkinson!' But he repeated 'Vilkinson?' It turned out that he was asking for razor blades. The only kind available in Hungary at that time was Russian soft steel razor blades which gave a very uncomfortable shave. Fortunately I had my Ladyshave with me and a few spare blades which we were able give to him and he was very grateful.

We swam in the Balaton where the shore is sandy and there are wooden steps that lead into the lake with a rail to hold on to so it is much easier than going for a swim in the sea. It was very warm at end of August.

One afternoon we went into a small grocery shop and suddenly we were face to face with my father's cousin Manyi whom I had not seen for over ten years. She looked at me in surprise and tentatively said, 'Zsuzsi? Is that you?' hardly believing her eyes. She had been banished to the country with so many others who lost their homes in Budapest in the 50's. She was with her second husband whom she nicknamed Pluto, a doctor who worshiped the ground Manyi walked on. She was the daughter of a doctor Moller from my father's side of the family and they were also on holiday in *Siófok*. It was a very happy reunion, we had much to talk about, but I lost touch with her again after we came back to England.

On Sunday I went to Mass in a little white-washed church full of old Hungarian women with their dark cotton weeds and head scarves. They sang in a mournful, wailing sort of way. 'Blessed Lady, Our Mother and Patroness, we call on you in our great need, remember Hungary, this corrupt land and the unfortunate people who live here,' and it made me cry to remember that I was also a Hungarian.

The following week, when we were back in Budapest, it rained a lot, but we were quite happy that the heat wave was over. The Palace Hotel on the *Rákoczi út* had an old time faded grandeur. There was a live group playing Hungarian folk music during dinner and the food was excellent. I asked one of the waiters to recommend a good cookery book that I could buy and purchased it. It was written by the chef called József Venesz who worked at that hotel. As our meals were included in the cost of the holiday it was not a very wise decision to accept an invitation to dinner by my uncle Cincó, but as it was my birthday I could not refuse. He was by then in a wheel chair because he was paralysed by a tumour on his spine but he was still working and we went to meet him in the flat originally owned by my grandmother Mucó. There was a restaurant opposite their house in Bajza utca 8 on the ground floor of a large block of flats built on the site of my old tennis court and ice rink and there I had the worst meal of my life! The potatoes must have been warmed up several times and tasted awful! I felt very sorry for Cincó who had his meals from here every day. His wife did not enjoy cooking and the restaurant had a take away option which was very reasonable. They were quite well off as he was a highly respected designer. Few people in those days could afford a car, let alone a Mercedes, like the one Cincó was driving! The only cars available were Trabants or Skodas and a 50% deposit was required to be placed on the waiting list for a car, and they still had to wait for a further four years.

We also visited my favourite uncle Feri who was suffering from bone cancer. He had survived the concentration camp and was well into his seventies. We arrived at the familiar flat in Kapás utca 49 and took the ancient elevator to the second floor. We were met by his wife Manci and my cousin Elly. Uncle Feri was lying on a settee in the living room and although he must have been in a great deal of pain he was smiling when he saw us. I was very pleased to be able to see him and introduce Michael to him and he was very happy to meet us. It was the last time I saw him as he died two weeks later.

We took some photographs of the statues at Heroes' Square and Anonymous, the famous historian whose statue is in the City Park, we visited Museums and the Castle with its many bullet holes from the 1956 revolution. Too soon it was time to return to England, for Michael, the University of East Anglia to complete his PhD, and for me the laboratories of Mackintosh's chocolate factory. Over the following years we returned to Budapest several times and noticed each time how much the living standards had improved.

On June 16, 1989 a huge crowd gathered to witness the fitting reburial of the martyrs of the 1956 revolution. Communism ended and the border was opened. On October 23, 1989 Hungary was renamed the Republic of Hungary and in the spring of 1990 - after 45 years of a single party regime - free elections were held.

In 1999 Hungary became a member of NATO and on 1 May 2004 Hungary became a member of the European Union.

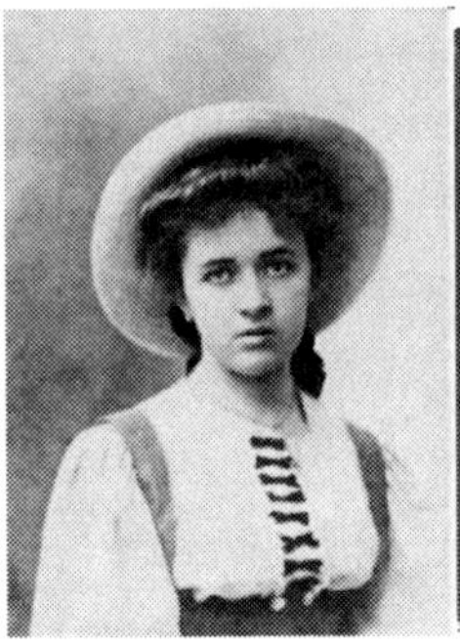

Margit before her marriage

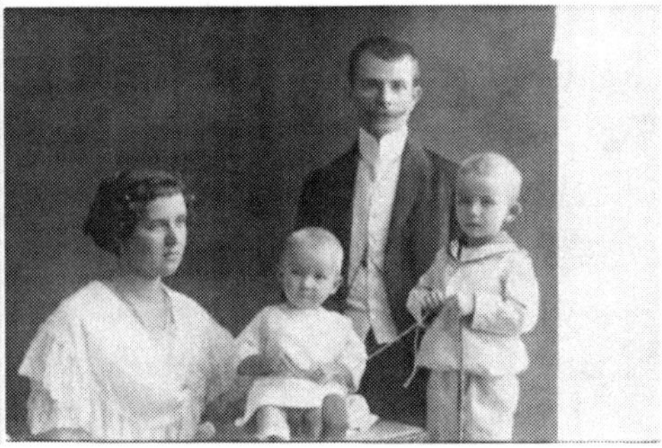

Bozzay family in 1913

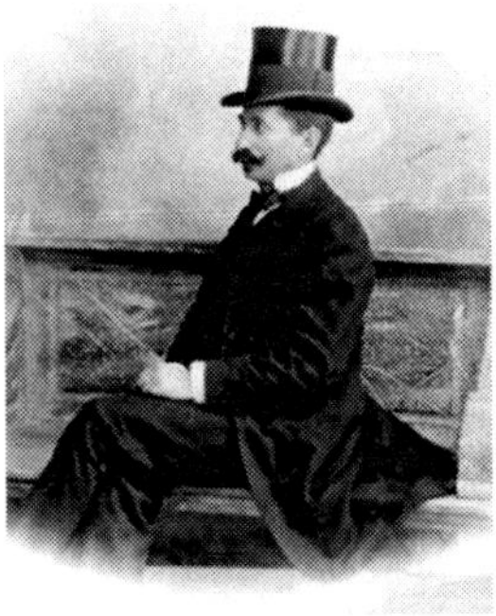

Vajda Adolf

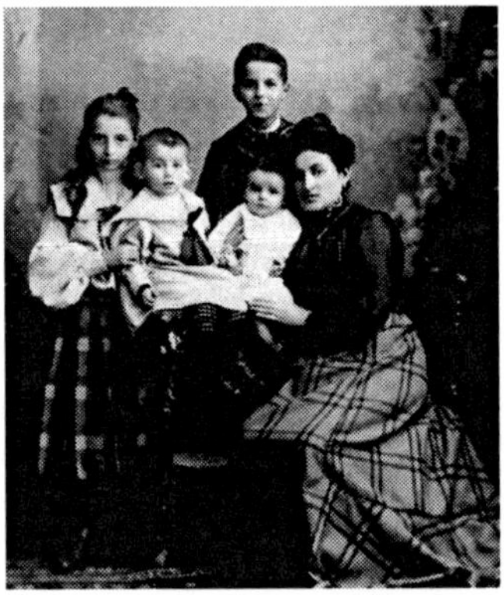

The Vajda family in 1905

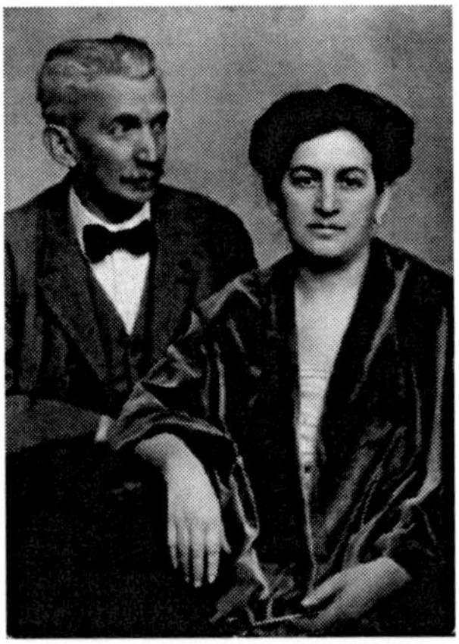

Vajda Adolf and Lotti

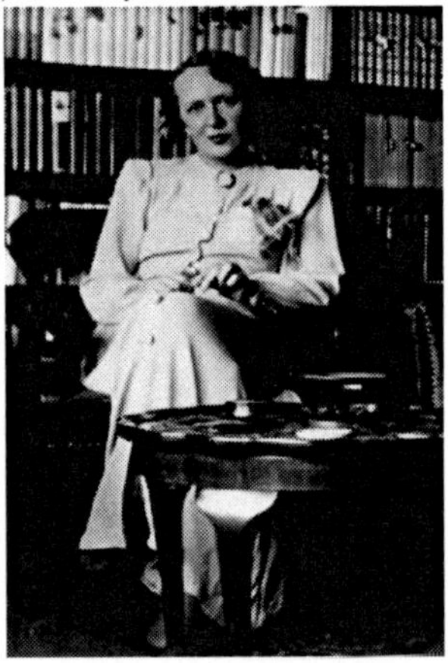

Bozzay Margit in 1941

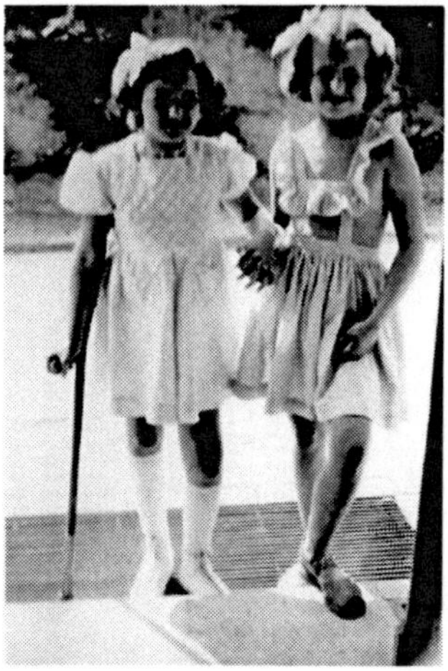

At the entrance to the flats with my friend Kerényi Judith in 1954.

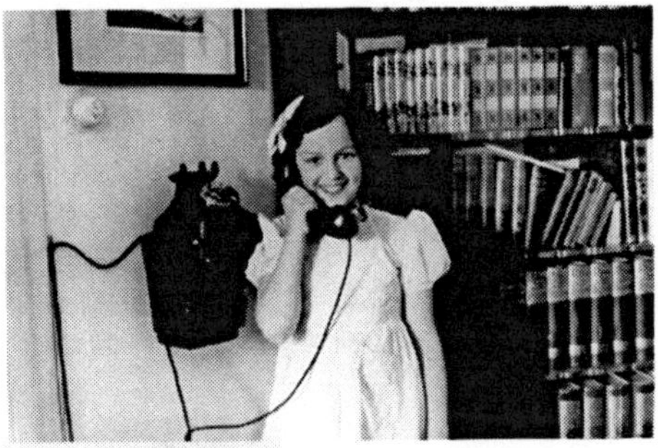

The book case and telephone in the flat.

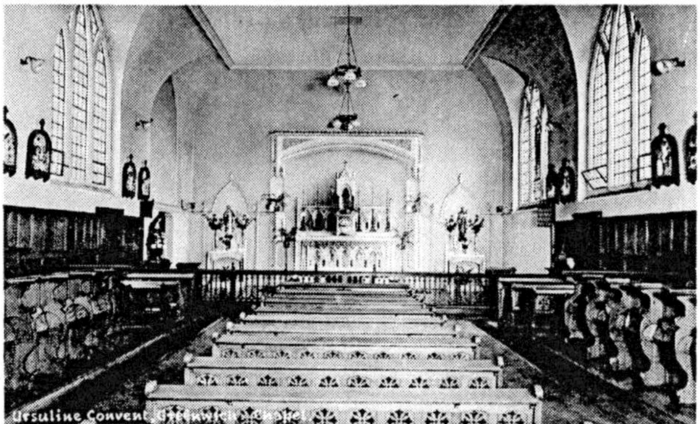

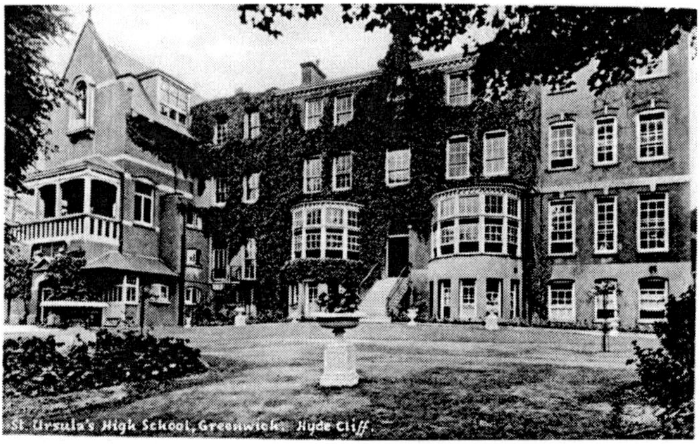

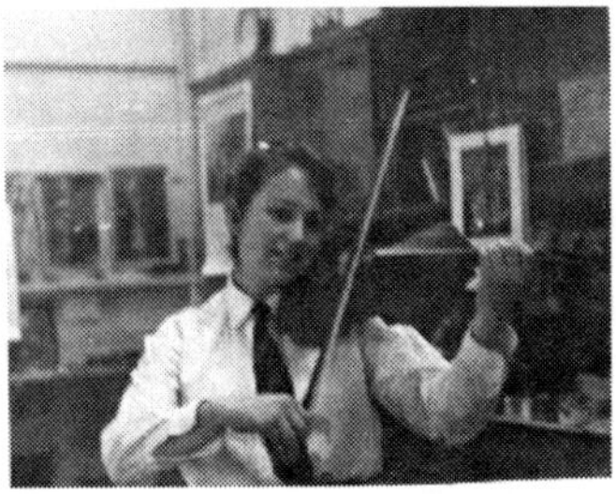

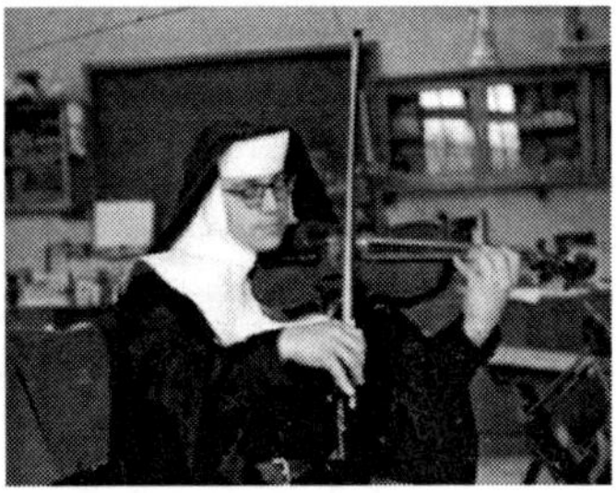

Playing the violin in the Art room with Mother Joan.

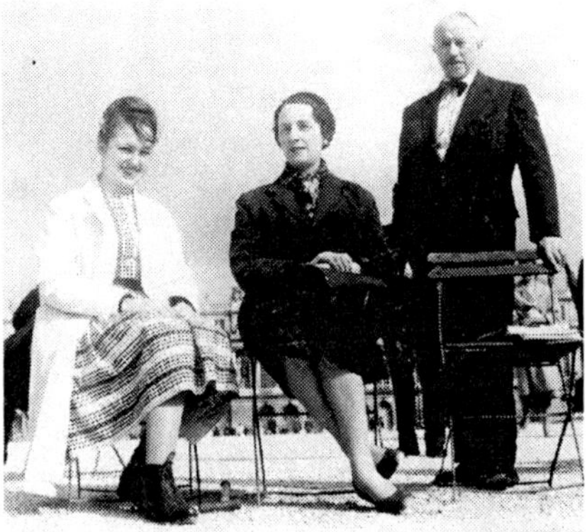

At Versaille with M. & Mme Poirrier in 1958

Lightning Source UK Ltd.
Milton Keynes UK
UKOW04f1204250913

217897UK00001B/30/P

9 781782 999683